Review of
Forensic Medicine

Seventh Edition

Review of
Forensic Medicine

Seventh Edition

Dr. Sumit Seth MBBS (MAMC), MD (LHMC)
INDIAN FOREIGN SERVICE

Ex-Senior Resident
Department of Forensic Medicine
Lady Hardinge Medical College and
Associated Smt. Sucheta Kriplani and
Kalawati Saran Hospital
New Delhi

PEEPEE
PUBLISHERS AND DISTRIBUTORS (P) LTD.®

Review of Forensic Medicine

Published by

Pawaninder P. Vij and Anupam Vij

Peepee Publishers and Distributors (P) Ltd.

Head Office: 160, Shakti Vihar, Pitam Pura
Delhi-110 034 (India)

Correspondence Address:

7/31, First Floor, Ansari Road, Daryaganj
New Delhi-110 002 (India)

Ph: 41512412, 23246245, 9811156083

e-mail: peepee160@yahoo.co.in

e-mail: peepee160@rediffmail.com

e-mail: peepee160@gmail.com

www.peepeepub.com

First Edition: **2005**
Seventh Edition: **2018**
Reprint: 2019

ISBN: 978-81-8445-244-0

Printed in India by Nutech Print Services - India

In memory of my dad,
the late Sh. Satish Kumar Seth,
who taught me the virtues of staying ahead of time and standing up against conventional wisdom

Read Less, Study More – But How ?

Introduction: The purpose of this book is to equip students with a robust study technique called Retro-Analysis.

Retro-Analysis ensures active learning and builds up "cognitive muscles" that help students separate confuzers (incorrect choices that resemble the correct answers) from correct answers, thereby providing the fundamental skills required for passing any multiple choice exam.

The One-Two-One Sandwich Regime: The best way to study this book, or any subject, is to follow this highly-rewarding study regime, where Retro-Analysis plays a central role. A student should study each topic, chapter, or module in three stages, creating a "sandwich" formation in terms of assigned time, where the ratio presents the sequence 1 : 2 : 1 for steps I, II and III, as described below:

I. **First Stage: Anterograde Reading** – a first sequential reading of the text.

II. **Second Stage: Retrograde Analysis*** (see below).

III. **Third Stage: Speed Revision** – reading the text again, along with your own handwritten/highlighted annotations.

For example, if it takes one hour of anterograde reading to cover a chapter, that first reading should be followed by two hours of retro-analysis of that chapter, followed further by a speed revision for one hour. This is known as One-Two-One Sandwich Regime.

What is Retro-Analysis?

Retro-Analysis is a reverse study technique, used not only for finding the correct answer, but also for understanding why the other three choices are wrong. This study technique involves adding handwritten annotations to the text to help create Concept Maps. Using MCQs as a yardstick, this means solving MCQs not by looking at the key but by actively seeking the correct answer. This is facilitated by reverse studying of the text of this book and any textbooks studied for graduation.

[**Statutory Warning:** The key given in the book has some deliberate! typos, so don't rely on it!]

Remember that the more closely the confuzer resembles the real answer, the **slipperier!** the MCQ, becomes.

Advantages of Retro-Analysis:

(1) Active learning;

(2) High retention and recall;

(3) Development of time-saving confuzer-spotting skills;

(4) Crystallising concept maps for long term memory vault;

(5) Prevention of careless errors in exams.

Conclusion: Once this Sandwich Study Regime becomes second nature, students will tread the path of great insight and gain decisive advantage vis-a-vis candidates who continue to Read More but Study Less. This is the Game-Changing Mantra, and I share it with you ::: *Read Less, Study More.*

Sumit Seth

e-mail: doctorsumitseth@gmail.com

@MedForensic

/ReviewFMT

Prologue

A bunch of class notes, scribbled in a manner which even trained pharmacists – accustomed to reading doctors' illegible handwriting – would find difficult to decipher, turned into a book, in 2004. The book was initially written off by some purists. Nonetheless, I wrote it as a labour of love. I was convinced that students needed a book like that. From the unassuming beginning of its first print, the book now has reached its seventh edition – spanning more than 14 years – and I'm humbled to discover that **#RoFM** ***has become a bestseller*** among books on Forensic Medicine on various online platforms.

I've revised the seventh edition with a deep sense of gratitude and responsibility. Along with some add-ons, I've written a new chapter, **'The Forensic Imaginarium',** in sync with the latest exam pattern of giving emphasis to images. Some portions of a few chapters have been rewritten, and newer concepts have been included. The chapter **'The Forensic Name Game'** captures the overarching theme of the book – *Read Less, Study More.* Well, in spite of my best efforts, I couldn't prevent the book from gaining a few extra pounds!

This book, RoFM, will help students understand and remember the important 'must knows' of Forensic Medicine. The focus is on assisting students grappling with information overload plus a need for rapid revision. With these ideas deliberated on, RoFM will help students grasp the essential areas of Forensic Medicine with ease. Please remember that **#RoFM** is **NOT a textbook but an enzyme!** with the singular aim of helping the content - from prescribed textbooks of Forensic Medicine – sift through a barrier normally difficult to cross, i.e., **the Blood-Brain Barrier.**

I've used my vast experience as a student and intensive knowledge as a teacher to ensure that the book ends up being 'reader friendly'. I have made my best effort to make this book complete yet concise. I request all readers to share your valuable suggestions for further improvement. In times when most books are written with 'the subject' in mind, I've written this book with 'the student' in mind.

I'm acutely aware that **'a good book cannot replace a good teacher'.** I'll keep tweeting and updating the FB page and interacting with you using the hashtag **#RoFM,** so that you don't miss out anything new and I can continue with my favourite hobby. In full disclosure, Forensic Medicine is no longer my active profession but a delightful avocation.

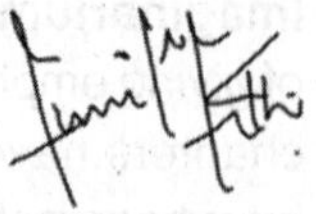

Sumit Seth

e-mail: doctorsumitseth@gmail.com

@MedForensic

/ReviewFMT

Acknowledgements

To my respected guide

Dr GK Sharma, Director Prof, Forensic Medicine, Ex-Principal and Medical Superintendent, Lady Hardinge Medical College, who has inspired me with his in-depth knowledge of the subject and his magnanimous personality. I'll always be indebted to him.

To my teachers

Dr Atul Murari and ***Dr Yashoda Rani***

who showed me the right way in life and taught me the intricacies of this subject.

To all my colleagues

for their help and cooperation in preparing the book.

To all my friends, especially

Dr Sumer Kumar Sethi (Radiologist) and ***Dr Vineet Malik*** (Cardiologist), for pushing me to take up this project and persevere with it. ***Dr Syeda Afshan and Dr Fahad Khan***, who read the previous edition with a *magnifying glass!* and sent me a list of errata, making the current edition typo free–almost!

Mr Pawaninder P Vij and Mr Anupam Vij (Publishers), without whose cooperation this book would never have been possible.

To my students of

Lady Hardinge Medical College (Hardonians), who showed faith in my ability as a teacher and constantly 'troubled me' with their never-ending queries.

To my virtual students

on Twitter, Facebook and Whatsapp!, all credits to them for keeping me and the knowledge of Forensic Medicine, on *my fingertips*– in this era of touch screen.

Special thanks to my younger brother, ***Amit,*** for letting me use the computer more than my fair share while I was writing the first edition (Those days, we had only one heavyweight desktop).

To my beloved wife, ***Tanu,*** for her love and support and also to our sons ***Shreshth and Saksham*** for providing a new meaning to our lives and *especially* for asking me numerous questions about Forensic Medicine and my book. An example: *"Why is there no digital edition of your book available, papa?"* Hmm!

Above all, to my mother, ***Smt. Urmil Seth***. What I've achieved is the outcome of her unconditional love and blessings.

Contents

1

Identification

- *Corpus Delicti:* Corpus delicti (body of offence, *essence of crime**) means, the elements of any criminal offence, e.g., murder.
- The main part of corpus delicti is the establishment of identity of the dead body.
- **Identification is established by the following data:**
  1. Race and religion
  2. Sex
  3. Age
  4. Stature
  5. Dactylography*
  6. Miscellaneous.

RACE

Race from skeletal remains.

Osteometery:

SKULL (the facial region) **most diagnostic*** for racial attribution.

- Cephalic Index = (Max breadth of skull/Max length of skull) × 100

  Cephalic Index was defined by Swedish professor of anatomy **Anders Retzius***

  Slide Callipers – used to measure the length and breadth of skull.

It **divides** skull into 3 categories:

- "**DuMB**" (Memorizer)

1. **Dolico-cephalic** (long-headed) **C.I.** 70 to 75
   – Seen in pure **Aryans**, Aborigines and Negroes.
   Anteroposterior diameter of skull is **MAX***.
2. **Mesaticephalic** (medium headed) **C.I.** 75 to 80
   – *Majority of Indians are mesaticephalic *(Not to confuse with CI of Aryans).*
3. **Brachycephalic** (short headed) **C.I.** 80 to 85
   – Seen in Mongoloids (maximum C.I.).
   Anteroposterior diameter of skull is **Minimum***

[Memorizer → **APe BRoMINe**]

Non-metric Racial Features of the skull – outlined by **Rhine*.**

The Negroid Skull
• **Post-Bregmatic Depression** • **Alveolar Prognathism**–the anterior protrusion of the alveolar process • **Guttered Nasal Sill** (most diagnostic feature of the Negroid face)

BONES OF UPPER LIMBS

- Brachial Index = (Length of Radius/Length of Humerus) × 100.

BONES OF LOWER LIMBS

- Crural Index = (Length of Tibia/Length of Femur) × 100
- For Indians Crural Index is **85 +/–2**
- Anterior Curvature of Femur is distinct in NEGROID race*
  {**N.B.** Intermembral Index = [(Length of Humerus +Radius)/Length of Femur + Tibia] × 100}.

Race from Hair

Negroids

- **MEDULLA IS FRAGMENTED*(N.B.: Some books "wrongly" mentioned non-**

fragmented medulla in Negroids including 6th edition of #RoFM)
- Kidney shaped cross-section
- Cuticle is absent*.

Caucasoids

- **MEDULLA IS FRAGMENTED***
- Oval shaped cross-section
- Cuticle is medium.

Mongoloids: **[Hair widest of the three races, Diameter is 100 microns or more]**
- **MEDULLA IS CONTINUOUS* (NON-FRAGMENTED)**
- Round in cross-section
- Cuticle is thick.

Race from Teeth

Negroids

Tuberculum Intermedium (extra lingual cusp)

*Caucasoids: [Memorizer→**C-CC**]*

Carbelli's **C**usps seen in (small nodule at lingual surface of molar in upper jaw).

Mongoloids

- **Largest teeth** among the 3 races
- **Third upper molar** Absent
- **Dens Evaginatus**–an extra tubercle on mandibular premolars
- **Protostylids**
- **Shovel** shaped incisor. Upper Central Incisor. Described by **Muhlrieter*(AIIMS May 17)**
- **Taurodontism** (Bull tooth)
- **Long pointed canine**
- **Enamel pearls.**

RELIGION

- Hindu females use **vermillion on head.**
- **Callosities** over forehead and lateral aspect of knees are useful to identify religion.

SEXUAL DIFFERENTIATION

Sex of an individual can be determined on the basis of:

- External features.
- Sex chromatin.
- Sexing of skeletal remains.

External Features

Most conclusive evidence lies is:
- The presence of ovaries in females.
- The presence of testis in males*.

Sex Chromatin

Sex from chromatin can be determined by:
- Barr body.
- Davidson-Smith body.
- Feulgen reaction.
- Quinacrine staining.

GONADAL BIOPSY

Confirmatory method of sex determination.

Barr Body

- Is a small planoconvex mass lying near nuclear membrane.
- **Barr body** was first demonstrated by **Barr and Bertam***.
- In buccal smear, it is present in 20 to 80% of cells in the female and 0 to 4% in males.
- The number of Barr bodies present is correlated with the formula: B = X–1 (B is the number of Barr bodies, X is the number of X chromosome).
- **Lyon's Hypothesis***: Barr body is inactivated X chromosome (Lyonization).
- **Buccal smear,** saliva, hair follicles are used in determination of sex.
- **Chromatin positivity:** 20-80% in females.

Davidson-Smith Body

- A small nuclear appendage of drumstick* form

(helps in sexing) present in Neutrophils in the female (6% of cells) but is absent in males.
Chromatin Positivity: 6% in females.

Feulgen Reaction

Acriflavin Schiff reagent is used to stain. X-chromosome, which is seen as bright yellow spot.
Chromatin Positivity: 50-70% in females.

Quinacrine Staining

The Y chromosome present in some cells demonstrate fluorescence, when stained with Quinacrine dihydrochloride.
Chromatin Positivity: 45-80% in males*.

INTERSEX

Definition

It is a condition in which characters of both sexes are present in varying degrees in one person including physical form, reproductive organs and sexual behaviour. It can be divided into **four groups:**

A. Gonadal Sex Disorder

1. **Gonadal agenesis**–In this, the testes or ovaries have never developed. The nuclear sex is negative.
2. **Gonadal dysgenesis**–External sexual structures are present, but at puberty, the testes or ovaries fails to develop.

B. Chromosomal Sex Disorder

a. **Klinefelter Syndrome**
   - The anatomical structure is male but the nuclear sexing is female.
   - The sex chromosome pattern is XXY (47 chromosomes).

		Male	Female
A. SKULL			
	Trait		
1.	General appearance	Larger, heavier, longer, prominent muscular markings. **Capacity:** 1500 to 1550 cc.	Smaller, smooth, rounder, lighter **Capacity:** 1350 to 1400 cc
2.	Architecture	Rugged	Smooth
3.	Forehead	Steeper, less rounded **[M]**	**Vertical, round*** [F]
4.	Glabella	More prominent	Less prominent
5.	Orbits	**Square,** relatively smaller	Rounded, relatively larger
6.	Supra orbital ridge	Prominent	Less prominent
7.	Cheek bones	Heavier, laterally arched	Lighter
8.*	**Frontal eminence**	Small*	**Large***
9.	Occipital area	Muscle lines and protuberance marked	Muscle line and protuberance not marked
10.	Mastoid process	Large, round, blunt	Small, smooth, pointed
11.	Palate	Larger, broader, tends more to U-shape	Small, tends more to parabola
12.	Foramina	Larger	Smaller
13.	Foramen magnum	Large and long	Relatively small and round
14.	Teeth	Larger	Smaller

Contd.

Contd.

		Male	*Female*
B.	**MANDIBLE**		
1.	General size	Larger and thicker	Smaller, thinner
2.	**Chin***	**Square**	**Rounded**
3.	Ascending ramus	Greater breadth	Smaller breadth
4.	Angle of body and ramus	Less obtuse (under 125°); prominent, everted	More obtuse; not prominent, inverted
5.	Condyles	Larger	Smaller
C.	**PELVIS**		
1.	Bony framework	Massive, rougher, marked muscle sites, narrow, tough	Less massive, smoother
2.	General	Deep funnel	Flat bowl
3.	Ilium	Less vertical	More vertical, distance between iliac crest is less
4.	**Preauricular* sulcus (used for sex determination)**	**Not frequent, narrow, shallow**	**More frequent, broad and deep**
5.	Obturator foramen	Large, often **oval*** with base upwards	Small, triangular with apex forwards
6.	**Greater sciatic notch***	**Smaller, narrower, deeper**	**Larger, wider, shallower**

Contd.

Contd.

		Male	*Female*
7.	Subpubic angle or pubic arch	**V**-shaped, 70-75° and sharp	**U-shaped**, broader, more than 90° (obtuse)
8.	Pelvic brim or inlet	Heart shaped	Circular or elliptical, diameter longer
9.	Ischiopubic Index = (Pubic length in mm/Ischial length in mm) × 100 **WASHBURN INDEX**	73 to 94	91 to 115 (more in female)
10.	Sciatic notch Index = (Width of sciatic notch/Depth of sciatic notch) × 100	4 to 5	5 to 6 (more)
11.	Corpobasal index of sacrum	**More in male****	Less in female
D.	**THORAX**		
1.	General	Longer and narrower	Shorter and wider
2.	Sternum	Body longer and more than twice the length of the manubrium; breadth more. Length more than 149 mm	Shorter and less than twice the length of the manubrium; breadth less, length less than 149 mm (**Ashley's rule**)*
3.	Sternal Index = (Length of manubrium/Length of body) × 100	46.2	54.3 (more in female)
4.	Ribs	Thicker, less curvature and are less oblique	Thinner, greater curvature, more oblique
5.	Clavicle	Longer, broader, heavier and less curved	More curved

- It is chromatin positive.
- Characterised by extensive fibrosis and **hyalinization of the seminiferous tubules**, and hyperplasia of Leydig cells.
- There is a delay in onset of puberty, behavioral disorders and mental retardation.

Diagnosis:

i. **Karyotyping:** Using lymphocytes/fibroblasts/aminocytes/chorionic villi.

ii. **XIST:** Presence of RNA for X-inactive-specific transcriptase.

b. Turner's Syndrome

- The anatomical structure is female but the nuclear sexing is male.
- The sex chromosome pattern is XO (45 chromosomes).

c. True hermaphroditism (Ovotesticular Disorder): In this an ovary and testis or two ovotestes are present within the external genitalia of both sexes.

C. Phenotypic Sex Disorder

Pseudohermaphroditism: Internally gonadal tissue of only sex is seen, but external appearance is of the opposite sex.

- **Male Pseudo-Hermaphrodite**
  - Nuclear sex–Male
  - Anatomical sex–Female
  (Testicular Feminisation)
- **Female Pseudo-Hermaphrodite**
  - Nuclear sex–Female
  - Anatomical sex–Male
  - Most common cause: Adrenal hyperplasia due to 21-hydroxylase deficiency.

{NB→***Colonel Victor Barker's Case**** was a famous case for **Concealed Sex**}

Krogman's Table*

%age of accuracy in determination of sex from bone.

Pelvis	95%
Skull	90-92%
Long Bones	80%
Pelvis + Skull	98%
All 206 bones	**100%**

- **Best bone for determination of sex is *Pelvis* (Phenice method** is used for the estimation of sex of an individual from the pelvis.)
- **Chilotic line** is useful in determination of **sex***
  - **Males→Sacral** part of **Chilotic line** more **prominent (MS degree!! Chill).**
  - Females→Pelvic part of Chilotic line more prominent.
- **Best criteria in pelvis to determine sex from pelvis is *Sciatic notch index**.***
- **Greater Sciatic Notch is L-shape in female (N.B.→ J-shape in male).**
- **Pre-Auricular Sulcus is a *Tertiary sexual characteristic*.**
- ***Corporo-Basal Index* is more in Males* (cf. with other indexes).**
- **Ashley's Rule** deals with differentiation of **sex using Sternum. (AIIMS Pre PG)**
- **Medullary Index = (Diameter of Medulla/ Diameter of whole bone) × 100, used for long bones (Most reliable Radius>Ulna>Tibia> Humerus).**

AGE

Age can be determined from:

1. Secondary sexual characteristics
2. Teeth
3. Ossification of bones.

1. SECONDARY SEX CHARACTERS

Boys' and girls' sexual maturity stage was assessed using **Marshal and Tanner criteria.**

In Males

- The first **SECONDARY SEX CHARACTERS 2 appear**

  Testes – large, firmer

  Penis – begins to enlarge

  Sequence of development of secondary sexual characters in male is

  ↑ size of testes

  ↓

  Adrenarche

  ↓

  Penile growth

  ↓

  Appearance of pubic hairs

  ↓

  Growth spurt (**occurs later in males and is of greater magnitude than in females**)

  ↓

  Moustache

  ↓

  Axillary hairs/Beard

In Females

- At 13-14 years–**breast begins to develop,** hair on mons veneris.
- Visual inspection of the vagina to assess estrogen stimulation.
  - Non-stimulated mucosa—glistening red*.
  - Stimulated mucosa—pinkish (**Estrogen–Pink**).
- Sequence of development of secondary sexual characters in females.

T→P→AGe→M

Thelarche (Beginning of breast development **Stage 1** Papilla elevation only).

↓

Pubarche

↓

Adrenarche

↓

Growth spurt

↓

Menarche

↓

Axillary hair

- Clinical condition in which secondary sexual characters appear earlier than average age is **McCune Albright syndrome.***
- Precautious puberty, 5 times **more common in girls (Most common cause idiopathic).**
- Appearance of Breast in **Males** (Gynaecomastia)
  - **C**imetidine
  - **T**estosterone
  - **S**pironolactone
  - **C**annabis
  - **A**lcohol
  - **N**ifedipine (CT SCAN)
- Conditions resulting in Hirsuitism
  - Stein Leventhal syndrome.
  - Bilateral polycystic ovaries.

2. TEETH

- Temporary or deciduous teeth are 20 in number–4 incisors, 2 canines and 4 molars in each jaw.
- In ill-nourished children and in **rickets, dentition** may be delayed.
- Dental aging may be the **most precise method** of age estimation, before the **age of 15 years.**
- In **Syphilis,** dentition appears early or, even present at birth (Hutch**IN**son-Boeck teeth-**IN**cisor).

- Mottle Teeth – Fluorosis.
- Fournier's Teeth – Syphilis, Permanent Molars.
- Eruption of temporary teeth is for 2 to 2½ years.
- The temporary teeth begins to fall at about the sixth or seventh year after eruption of first permanent molar.
  - In children, mixed dentition* (temporary + permanent) remains at 6-12 years of age.The total no. of teeth remains 24*.
  - PALMER NOTATION is more commonly used in India.
- **Difference between Temporary and Permanent teeth:**

	Trait	*Temporary teeth*	*Permanent teeth*
1.	Size	Smaller, lighter, narrow	Heavier, stronger, broader
2.	Crown	**China-white color (CT)**	**Ivory-white color (IP)**
3.	Neck	More constricted	Less constricted
4.	Ridge	A ridge or thick edge at the junction of crown with the fangs present (between root and fin)	No ridge**

- **Calcification and Eruption of Deciduous Teeth:** The sequence of eruption of temporary teeth is memorised as **"IaM-CM" (Memorizer).**

Tooth		*Eruption*
1. Central Incisor		
a. Lower (oldest)	(a)	6-8 months **(6 months)**
b. Upper	(b)	7-9 months **(7 months)**
2. Lateral Incisor		
a. Upper	(a)	7-9 months **(8 months)**
b. Lower	(b)	10-12 months **(9 months)**
3. First Molar		12-14 months **(12 months)**
4. Canine		17–18 months **(12 + 6 = 18 months)**
5. Second molar (youngest)		20-30 months **(24 months)**

- **Calcification and Eruption of Permanent Teeth:** Sequence of eruption of permanent teeth is memorised as: '**M**arry **I**s **I**n **P**ain **P**eter **C**an **M**ake **M**edicine'.

Tooth	Eruption	Permanent*	Temporary
1. First Molar **(M) - Oldest**	6-7 years (6 yrs)	4	20
2. Central Incisor **(I)**	6-8 years (7 yrs)	8	16
3. Lateral Incisor **(I)**	8-9 years (8 yrs)	12	12
4. First pre Molar **(P)**	9-10 years (9 yrs)*	16	8
5. Second pre Molar **(P)**	10-11 years (10 yrs)	20	4
6. Canine **(C)**	11-12 years (11 yrs)	24	0
7. Second Molar **(M)**	12-14 years (13 yrs)	28	
8. **Third Molar*** (M) **- Youngest**	**17-25 years (18 yrs)**	**32**	

(*Most erratic in eruption, DEMIRJIAN METHOD (orthopantomograms) is the most suitable method for estimating age using Third molar)

*[Short Cut→Total permanent teeth= (Age-5) × 4]

Superadded Teeth: All permanent molars are superadded teeth, i.e., they come directly without any predecessor. Total 12.

Successional Teeth: All permanent teeth which come in place of temporary teeth are successional Teeth. Total 20.

Supernumerary Tooth: A supernumerary tooth is one that is additional to the normal series. The most common is maxillary incisor* **(Mesiodens).**

Distodens are supernumerary molars.

Spacing of Jaw: After eruption of 2nd molar, the ramus of mandible grows to create space for the 3rd molar.

'Twelve-year-old tooth': Second Molar, which erupts between 12 and 13 years of age.

Gustafson's Method (ex-vivo method)

The age estimation of adult over 25 years (between 25 and 60 years) depends on the physiological age changes in each of the dental tissue. The various criteria used in Gustafson's method is ***'SCRIPT'***: (Memorizer)

S – Secondary Dentine
C – Cementum Apposition
R – Root Resorption
Attr**I**tion
P – Paradentosis (Estimated before tooth extraction)

T – Translucency* → (The most reliable criterion of Gustafson's method)

- Gustafson's method is a **postmortem*** procedure.
- Translucency is seen after 30 years of age.
- Anterior teeth are more suitable than posterior.
- Merit of this method decreases from incisors to premolars.
- 3rd molar is least preferred.
- Error increases after 50 years.

Daliz Method is a modification of Gustafson's method (root resorption and cementum apposition are NOT considered).

Lamendil's Method

Estimation of age from teeth (**Postmortem*** procedure) using 2 criteria:

- Gingival Recession.
- Root Transparency.

Boyde's Method

Estimation of ***Age from Teeth*** by counting ***Incremental Lines**** in histological section.

Nolla Method (enN-vivo)

Nolla classified dental development into 10 calcification stages from crypt state to closure of the root apex. Mineralization and development begins and ends earlier in females, the sequence of development finalization remains same in both males and females. The Nolla method is one of the most widely used clinically as a reliable procedure for dental development estimation in **permanent teeth**.

Stack's Method

Stack evolved a method to know the age of **infants from the weight and height of the erupting teeth** of child.

Miles formula—Miles determined age at death by measuring the thickness of enamel and dentine from neonatal line and divided it by appropriate daily rate of formation.

Mineralization of deciduous dentition commences from **2-4 months in-utero**. Some of the histological methods can detect early mineralization **12 weeks** before being detectable in the radiographs.

The neonatal line is considered as an indicator of birth. Neonatal lines are present in both enamel and dentin of deciduous teeth and **permanent first molars** which indicate the development during the transitional period between intrauterine and extra uterine environments.

In the dentin:

- **Incremental lines of Von Ebner**.
- **Contour lines of Owen** are present.

These lines are used to estimate age of the neonates or foetus at death.

Incremental lines of Retzius are caused by variation in the rhythmic mineralization of enamel prisms:

Incremental lines are also produced by:
- Tetracycline
- Lead
- Strontium
- Fluoride incremental lines.

Orthopantomography (OPT) is the method of choice to evaluate the development of each of the teeth using radiographic records also known as **Panoramic Radiography.**

Dental Examination best way to identify bodies in **Mass Disaster. (CET 2016)**

Charting of Teeth

1. **Universal system:** Each teeth is given a number 1 through 16 for upper jaw, beginning from right upper third molar and 17 through 32 for lower jaw, beginning from left lower third molar.

2. **Palmer's system:** The teeth of each quadrant are numbered from 1 to 8, beginning with central incisor and moving away from midline.
3. **Haderup system:** Similar to Palmer's notation, except that it uses + sign for upper teeth and a – sign for lower teeth. The sign is placed before the number for left teeth and after the number for right teeth.
4. **Federation Dentuire Internationale (FDI):** Two digit system. It is similar to Palmer, but substitute a number for quadrant sign. 1 for right upper, 2 for left upper, 3 for left lower and 4 for right lower quadrant.
5. **Zigmondy's method:** This is similar to Palmer's method. The teeth of each quadrant are numbered from 1 to 8, beginning with central incisor and moving away from midline. In this method roman numbers are used for deciduous teeth.

PQZ – Potential Question Zone
How to denote Lower Left Canine?
1. Universal : 22
2. Palmer : 3 Lower Left
3. Haderup : (-)3L

Chemical Analysis

- Nitrogen content of enamel increases with age.
- Concentration of copper, selenium, lead and iron ions increases with age.
- Carbonate content *decreases* with age.
- **Aspartic Acid Racemization:** Aspartic acid racemization in teeth enamel provides a bio-chronological tool for assessing the age.

Preservation of Bite Mark

- Bite marks on deceased victim's **Skin** is preserved in **Formalin**.
- Bite mark on fruits–**Campden** Fruit Preserving Solution which contains **Potassium or Sodium Metabisulfite.**

3. BONE AGE

There are 3 methods of determining bone age:

1. **Quantitative methods:** X-rays of half of the skeleton; are very penetrating; not often used.
2. **Qualitative methods:**
   i. ***Greulich and Pyle Atlas is the best*** known for qualitative method. It is based on frontal left-hand wrist and palm X-rays. Morphological variation of centers of ossification for a given articulation, and comparison to pictures of atlas of reference.
   ii. ***Taner and Whitehouse method*** (TW3) is based on frontal **left-hand wrist and palm** X-rays. It is a specific study of each bone to evaluate the development of certain hand and wrist bones.
   iii. ***Sauvegrain and Nahum method*** is based on scoring **elbow bones**.
   iv. ***Risser test*** is based on a study of the development of the **iliac crest points** of ossification from a frontal view of the pelvis.
3. **Index methods:** Numerical score given for each step of ossification. Scores are added up to a total number to determines level of ossification.

Memory Box
Greulich and Pyle method (GP) vs. Taner and Whitehouse method*(TW3) GP more rapid and easy to learn and **most often used.** TW3 is time consuming difficult to learn, best correlation to chronological age hence **more accurate** and offers better reproducibility.

Growth in Individual Bones

Age	*Bone centers*
11th week IUL	806
Birth	450
Adults	206

- **Union of epiphyses** in cartilaginous bone occurs by about **1 year earlier in female** than in male, **but opposite** is seen in suture closure of the skull. **The most studied anatomical region for age diagnosis (before 18 years): Carpus and the Hand.**
- The **pubic symphysis** is **the best single** criterion for determining age from 2nd to 5th decades.*
- **Sternum:** The four pieces of the body of the sternum fuse with one another **from below upwards*** between 14 and 25 years.
  At about 40 years, the **xiphoid** unites with the body. The manubrium fuses with the body at **old age.**
- **Hyoid**
  - The greater cornu of the hyoid bone unites with the body between 40 and 60 years.
- **Skull**
  1. The anterior fontanelles close and the two halves of the mandible unite at the **second year. Metopic suture *closes at 2-4 years may extend to 6 years.**
  2. The basi-occipital fuses with the basi-sphenoid at **about 18 to 21 years.**
  3. In the vault of the skull, union occurs in the inner table of skull 5 to 10 years **earlier** than on the outer tables.
  4. Closure of coronal suture starts at the age of **30-35** years.
  5. Closure of all sutures indicates age **more** than 60 years.
  6. The most successful estimate of age is done **is Sagittal Suture followed by Lambdoid then Coronal.**
  7. Masto-Occipital Suture is the **last to close***.
  8. Lateral Head Skiagram is used to observe skull sutures.
  9. **Closure:** Lambda (6 weeks), Pterion and Asterions (4 months), Bregma (18 months).

Sacrum: The sacrum becomes a single bone between 20 and 25 years.

Mandible:

A. **Angle of Mandible:** In **old age and children*, ramus of mandible** makes obtuse angle with the body about 140 degrees. **[Short Cut→ORO*, i.e., Obtuse (Child) Right (Adult) Obtuse (Old)].**

B. **Mental Foramen:** It moves towards Alveolar Margin with Age.

C. **Shape of Chin:** Sex Determination (**Males Square** and Females Round).

- **X-rays–Age Determination**

Age	*X-rays*
1. 13-16 years	1. Pelvis 2. Elbow
2. 13 years	Centers in triradiate cartilage of acetabulum and lesser trochanter of femur
3. 14 years	Center for iliac crest, medial and lateral epicondyles fuse with trochlea, patella completely ossify
4. 15 years	Fusion of triradiate cartilage of acetabulum
5. 16 years	Centre for ischial tuberosity, fusion of lower end of humerus, olecranon to ulna, upper end of radius and ulna
6. 21 years	Fusion of ischial tuberosity and inner end of clavicle.

- **Fusion of Joints**
  - In females fusion occurs 1-2 years earlier* (Except skull, sutures obliterates earlier in males).
  - Ossification occurs earlier in tropical countries vis-a-vis temperate countries.
  - **Galstaun's standard charts** for Epiphyseal Union are widely used in India.

Joints	*Approximate age of fusion*
Shoulder joint	18 years
Elbow joint	16 years
Wrist joint	18 years
Hip joint	17-18 years
Knee joint	18 years
Ankle joint	16-17 years

Ossification	*Intrauterine life*
1. Centre for clavicle	2nd week* (1st centre)
2. Calcaneum	5th month
3. Sternum (2nd and 3rd piece of body)	7th month
4. Talus	7th month
5. Lower end of femur	10th lunar month/Birth
6. Upper tibia	Birth
7. Head of humerus	Birth

Ossification of the Carpal Bones

Predictable sequence
Starting with the **Capitate** and ending with the **Pisiform**. (C→P)
[Beware!→**CHaT + LuST = TraP]**

- Capitate: 2 months (first*)
- **Ha**mate: 3 months
- **T**riquetrum: 3 years
- **Lu**nate: 4 years
- **S**caphoid: 5 years
- **T**rapezium: 6 years
- **Trap**ezoid: 7 years

- **P**isiform: 8-12 years (last)

- **Age rule of Palm!** → Between 2-6 years number of carpal bones present on X-ray represent approximately age.
- 1st ossification centre to appear: **Clavicle and lower jaw** at **2nd week** of intrauterine life.
- Dental age is a more accurate index for age estimation for the early teens.
- Bone age, **except the clavicle**, allows estimation until 18 years.

Age of the Foetus

Rule of Haase

- A rough method of calculating the age of the foetus.
  1. **Upto 5 months,** age of foetus = $\sqrt{\text{length}}$ (in cm).

Medicolegal Importance of Age

Age	*Medicolegal Aspect*	*Indian Penal Code/Acts Importance*	*Explanation*
12 weeks (IUL)	One doctor can do MTP		
20 weeks (IUL)	Only Therapeutic MTP possible		
> 7 months (IUL)	Infanticide	Sec. 300 IPC	Viability
> 5 years	Criminal Responsibility	Railways Acts	Punishability
> 7 years	Criminal Responsibility	Sec. 82 IPC	No criminal intent
10 years	Kidnap Child	Sec. 369 IPC	Rob movable property
Between 7 and 12 years	Criminal Responsibility	Sec. 83 IPC	Guilty of offence
> 12 years	Consent for non-invasive procedure	Sec. 89 IPC	Less than 7 years parents/guardian give consent for non-invasive procedure (12-18 years person can give consent)
< 14 years	Employment	Factory's Act	Cannot be employed
14-15 years	—Do—	—Do—	Employed with fitness certificate
> 15 years	—Do—	—Do—	Employment with fitness certificate
< 15 years (girls)	Rape	Sec. 375 IPC	Sexual intercourse with wife without consent
< 16 years (boys)	Kidnapping	Sec. 361 IPC	Taking away without the consent from lawful guardian

Contd.

Contd.

Age	*Medicolegal Aspect*	*Indian Penal Code/Acts Importance*	*Explanation*
< 18 years (girls)	Statutory rape*	**Sec. 375 IPC (changed in 2013)**	Sexual intercourse with girl with or without consent
< 18 years (girls)	Kidnapping	Sec. 361 IPC	Taking away without the consent from lawful guardian
< 18 years (girls)	Kidnapping	Sec. 366-A of IPC	Procuring a girl for illicit intercourse
> 18 years	Consent	Sec. 87 IPC	Consent for invasive procedure
> 18 years	Majority attainment	Sec. 3 Indian Majority Act, 1875	Testamentary Capacity Valid will, adult franchise (Voting)
> 18 years (girls)	Marriage	Child Marriage Restraint Act	—
> 16 years	Adult Judicial Punishment	Juvenile Justice Act 2000*	Boys and girls above 18 are Adult under Special Circumstances
< 21 years (girls)	Kidnapping	Sec. 366-B of IPC	—
> 21 years	Attainment of majority	Sec. 3 Indian Majority Act	Under guardianship of courts
> 21 years (boys)	Marriage	Child Marriage Restraint Act, 1978-79	—
25 years	Contesting Lok Shaba election Consuming alcohol in restaurants and bars	People's Representation Act	—
30 years	Contesting Rajya Sabha election	—Do—	—
35 years	Presidential elections	—	—
60 years	Employment	—	Age of retirement

2. **> 5 months** = (length (in cm)/5) = months (**Morrison's* modification of Hasse's Rule**).

1. **End of 3rd month**
   1. Foetus 7.5-10 cm long.
   2. Limbs are well developed.
   3. Neck is formed.
   4. Finger toes visible.
      (Sex can be determined in fetus after end of 4th month)*.
2. **End of 5th month**
   1. Foetus 17.5–20 cm long.
   2. Eyebrows are absent.
   3. Meconium is present in the stomach.
3. **End of 7th month**
   1. Length 35 cm.
   2. Weight 0.9 to 1.2 kg.
   3. Nails are thick.
   4. Eyelids open and papillary membrane disappears.
   5. Meconium is found in entire large intestine.
   6. Testes are found at **external** inguinal ring.
   7. Placenta weighs 350-400 gm.
   8. Vernix caseosa is present.
4. **End of 8th month**
   1. Length 40 cm.
   2. Nails reach the tips of finger.
   3. Left testis is present in the scrotum.
   4. Placenta weighs **500 gm**.
5. **End of 9th month**
   1. Length 45 cm.
   2. Scrotum is wrinkled and **contains both testes.**
   3. Placenta **weighs 500 gm.**
6. **End of 10th month (full term child)**
   1. Length **50-53 cm.**
   2. Crown-rump length **30-33 cm.**
   3. Weight **2.5-5 kg.**
   4. Lanugo absent except on shoulder.
   5. Testes are present in **scrotum.**

6. The center of ossification is found for **lower** end of femur.
7. Nails extend beyond the finger tips at the end of 40 weeks.

Stature

Stature from long bones can be estimated using regression formulae, some of the popularly used formulae are:

1. **Karl-Pearson***
2. Trotter and Glessor
3. Dupertius and Hadden
4. Jit and Singh.

Geneva Agreement deals with the reconstruction of the stature with the aid of the long bones.

Hepburn Osteometric Board – used to measure stature.

Multiplication factors for different bones are: {Short cut→***add. 0.8*** after multiplication factor of Femur, i.e., 3.7* in this sequence Fe-THUR.

Long bones of lower limbs more reliable

Bones	*Multiplication factor*
Radius	6.5(6.1+.8/2)
Ulna	6.1(5.3+.8)
Humerus	5.3(4.5+.8)
Tibia/Fibula	4.5(3.7+.8)
Femur	**3.7**

Most accurate estimate of stature : Femur > Tibia > Humerus > Radius

Dactylography (Fingerprint system, Galton system, Dermatoglyphycs)

- Most reliable* method of identification of a person.
- First used by **William Herschel**, he established the **First Fingerprint Bureau*** at *Writer's Building, Calcutta*, India.*
- Fingerprints are impressions of pattern formed by the papillary ridges of the fingertips.

- Fingerprint identification is based on two basic **Axioms:**
  1. **Persistence or Immutability**–The basic characteristics of fingerprints do not change with time.
  2. **Individuality**–The fingerprint is unique to an individual. The pattern is **different even in identical twins (Adolphe Quetelet's Rule*** ***of biological variation*****).**
- The patterns are not inherited. Fingerprint ridge pattern begin to develop at 16 weeks (IUL), fully developed by 25 weeks (IUL).
- Sequence of Ridge Pattern: Finger tips –> Palms –> Soles.

Fingerprints are **classified** primarily as:
1. **Loops 67% (most common*)**
   PQZ: Left Loops (35%) more common than Right Loops (32%)
2. **Whorls (29%)**
3. **Arches**
4. **Composite forms–1-2% (least common*)**.

- **Minutiae** are the principal features used to compare two fingerprints. Locard established the first rules for the minimum number of minutiae necessary for identification.

Elements of A Fingerprint

- **Delta:** When ridges converge on a point from three directions, the point is called delta. Outermost point of a ridge pattern.
- **Core:** The central area of the pattern is called the core.
- **Recurve:** A recurve is any ridge retracing its course.
- The 2 most widely used Chemical Reagents for fingerprint collections are:
  a. Ninhydrin.
  b. Cyanoacrylate.

- **Pigeon Hole Method** is manual method to record fingerprints.
- **FINDER** is a fingerprints recording software used by FBI, US – little finger is EXCLUDED, 8 fingers are recorded.
- **O-FTIR:** Optical Frustrated Total Internal Reflection (FTIR) is most commonly used to capture live scan fingerprints.
- In India, left **thumb impression is taken in males** and right thumb in females (Reasoning: Most males do manual work with right hand so may have injury scar).

Fingerprint Classification

A. Ten print classification
B. Single print classification
  - Henry System
  - Battley Systems (best known system).

Categories of Fingerprints

- **Latent Fingerprints**→Barely visible. Can be made visible by treating them with 5% **Silver Nitrate and fixed with 1% Sodium Thiosulfate [PQZ].**
- **Plastic Fingerprints**→Prints made on soft surface (Soap, cheese etc).
- **Visible Fingerprints**→Stained with blood, greese etc.
- **In *Leprosy, Charring, Radiation injury, Exposure to Dry Ice (CO_2),* fingerprints may be lost*.**

Fingerprints and Law

a. **Art. 20(3)–Constitution of India:** No person accused of any offence shall be compelled to be a witness against oneself.
b. **Sec. 73 Indian Evidence Act, 1872:** The Court may direct any person present in Court to prove fingerprint expressions.

c. **Mohan Lal vs. Ajit Singh Case:** Supreme Court ruled that minimum number of points/Minutiae to establish a proof of identity is **8*(ATE).**

Other Important Methods Used in Identification

1. **Poroscopy**—This is the further study of fingerprints utilizing study of pores was described by *Edmund Locard (Locard also is famous for Exchange Principle).*
2. **Chelioscopy***—The study of furrows and grooves present in human lips. **Suzuki** devised the classification system for lip prints.
3. **Rugoscopy**—**Harrison Allen** suggested use of human palatal rugae as a method of identification. Palate prints are taken from **anterior 1/3rd.**
4. **Podogram** is used for footprints.
5. **Bertillion System** ***(Portrait Parle*)***—Anthropometric system based on the physical measurement of specified parts of body, ***even if there are no biological specimens*.***
6. **Superimposition:**
   A technique in identifying a person by superimposing the X-ray of **skull** found after death on the **photo of his face of the person.**
   A negative result having more credibility because it can definitely be stated that the skull and the photograph are not those of the same person.
7. **Tattoo Marks:**
   - Dyes used: India Ink, Prussian Blue, Vermillion, Cinnabar.
   - Faded tattoo mark become visible by ultraviolet lamp.
   - Infrared photography makes old tattoo visible.
   - Tattooing of old decomposed body can be visualised by UV rays, IR rays, 3% Hydrogen Peroxide, Magnifying glass.
   - **Sydney Shark Arm case** identification was done by tattoo marks.

Methods to Erase Tattoo

- **B**urning and scarring.
- **B**eam (laser).
- **C**orrosives and caustic chemicals, e.g., Glycerin + Papain.
- **D**ry ice.
- **E**lectrolysis.
- **E**xcision and graft.

8. **X-ray Frontal Sinus:**
   - Useful in individuals > 15 years, when antemortem X-ray is available.

HAIR

Human Hair

- Fine, thin, **cuticular scales** are short, broad, not continuous; **cortex–thick,** 4-10 times as broad as medulla; **medulla–thin,** pigment–evenly distributed.
- **Precipitin test*** is specific **for human beings.**

Animal Hair

- Coarse, thick, cuticular scales very large, step like projection; **cortex–thin.**

Some Important Facts

- **Blood groups** can be determined in a **hair** from any part of the body by a **modified absorption elution technique.**
- **Chronological order of appearance of hair** Pubic Hair→Moustache→Beard/Axillary Hair.
- Scalp hair grow at **3** mm a week.
- Hair becomes loose after **72 hours** of death.

Age Determination of Scars

Duration	*Features*
5-6 days	Reddish/blue, firm union.
2 weeks-2 months	Pale, soft and sensitive. Tenderness +
2-6 months	Brown, tough, glistening. Tenderness mild
> 6 months	White, tough, non-tender.

Identification of Human Remains

- Amino acid racemization (e.g. Aspartic acid).
- Blood grouping.
- DNA analysis.
- Magnesium/Zinc ratio.
- Incremental lines in 2nd molar (Maple).

MCQs

1. **In Gustafson's method of age determination from teeth, the most reliable criterion is:**
   A. Cementum opposition
   B. Root reabsorption
   C. Secondary dentile deposition
   D. Root transparency
2. **The basi-occipital bone fuses with basi-sphenoid between:**
   A. 15 and 16 years **B.** 18 and 20 years
   C. 24 and 25 years **D.** 50 and 54 years
3. **Most reliable identification method used by police to identify criminal is:**
   A. Photography
   B. Galton's system
   C. Bertillon system
   D. Superimposition method
4. **Locards method of identification means:**
   A. Dactylography
   B. Poroscopy
   C. Anthropometry
   D. Cheiloscopy (lip prints)
5. **Ridges on the fingertips are detected upto the depth of:**
   A. 0.4 mm **B.** 0.6 mm
   C. 0.8 mm **D.** 1 mm
6. **Callosities present on the forehead of person indicate his:**
   A. Sex **B.** Race
   C. Religion **D.** Age

1 D 2 B 3 B 4 B 5 B 6 C

7. **Age of a scar when it is white glistening and tough is:**
   A. 1 week to 2 weeks
   B. 2 weeks to 1 month
   C. 1 month to 2 months
   D. 3 months to 6 months
8. **Shovel shaped incisor tooth is seen in:**
   A. Negroes **B.** Aryan
   C. Europeans **D.** Chinese
9. **Thickness of cortex of human hair in comparison to medulla is:**
   A. Half **B.** Same
   C. 2-3 times **D.** 5-10 times
10. **Fetal parts can be detected on X-ray examination in foetus of:**
    A. 8 weeks **B.** 12 weeks
    C. 16 weeks **D.** 20 weeks
11. **Sex can be accurately determined from long bones up to:**
    A. 95% **B.** 90%
    C. 85% **D.** 80%
12. **Crown Heal length of 6 months old fetus would be:**
    A. 20 cm **B.** 25 cm
    C. 30 cm **D.** 36 cm
13. **Least common type of fingerprints is:**
    A. Loop **B.** Arches
    C. Whorls **D.** Composite
14. **Pearson's formula is used to determine:**
    A. Sex **B.** Race
    C. Age **D.** Stature
15. **Minimum age of a person who can be punished under railway act is:**
    A. 3 years **B.** 5 years
    C. 7 years **D.** 12 years

---

7 D 8 D 9 D 10 C 11 D 12 C 13 D
14 D 15 B

16. **Normal adult male skeleton weighs approximately:**
A. 3.5 Kgm
B. 4.5 Kgm
C. 6.5 Kgm
D. 8.5 Kgm

17. **Greater sciatic notch in female is:**
A. Smaller
B. Wider
C. Narrower
D. Deeper

18. **Pre auricular sulcus is seen in:**
A. Ear
B. Skull
C. Pelvis
D. Femur

19. **Sex chromosome pattern in Klinefelter's syndrome is:**
A. XXY
B. XO
C. XX
D. XY

20. **Human skeleton is made up of:**
A. 106 bones
B. 126 bones
C. 206 bones
D. 226 bones

21. **Juvenile is a girl who has not attained the age of:**
A. 12 years
B. 14 years
C. 16 years
D. 18 years

22. **The age of a 16-year-old female is best determined by the radiograph of:**
A. Lower end of Radius and Ulna
B. Upper end of Humerus
C. Upper end of Radius and Ulna
D. Xiphisternum

23. **Legal age for marriage for boys in India:**
A. 18
B. 19
C. 20
D. 21
E. 25

24. **Most common pattern of fingerprint is:**
A. Arch
B. Loop
C. Whorl
D. Composite

16 B 17 B 18 C 19 A 20 C 21 D 22 C
23 D 24 B

25. Cephalic index is used for determination of:
A. Race
B. Age
C. Sex
D. Pelvic abnormality

26. Most reliable method of identification of a person is by:
A. Scars
B. Anthropometry
C. Fingerprinting
D. Photography

27. Pre-auricular sulcus is used for:
A. Determination of race
B. Determination of age
C. Determination of sex
D. None of the above

28. To determine the age of a 16-year-old girl which of the following is to be radiographed?
A. Wrist B. Knee
C. Ankle D. Elbow

29. Superimposition technique is used in:
A. Skull B. Pelvis
C. Femur D. Ribs

30. Second molar erupts at:
A. 6 years B. 12 years
C. 18 to 22 years D. 25 to 28 years

31. Tatoo is useful in identifying body *except*:
A. Living B. Dead
C. Decomposed D. Burnt

32. Best method for Identification of a person is by:
A. Scars
B. Blood group
C. DNA analysis
D. Fingerprints

25 A 26 C 27 C 28 D 29 A 30 B 31 D
32 D

33. To make a positive identification with the help of a partial finger point, the points of similarity should be at least:

A. 10 B. 12
C. 16 D. 20

34. Skull of a male differs from that of a female by all of the following *except:*

A. Capacity greater than 1500 c.c.
B. Muscular markings over occipital bone are less marked
C. Orbits square
D. Frontal eminence small

35. True about human hair is:

A. Medulla is 1/3rd or cortex
B. Cortex is 1/3rd of medulla
C. Has scales
D. None of the above

36. The average length of a full term child will be about:

A. 30 cms B. 35 cms
C. 40 cms D. 50 cms

37. When any two objects come into contact there is always a transference of material from each object on to the other. This is called:

A. Locard's exchange principle
B. Corpus delicti
C. Metallic fouling
D. Rule of Haase

38. Crown-heel length of five months foetus would be:

A. 16 cm
B. 25 cm
C. 30 cm
D. 35 cm

33 C 34 B 35 C 36 D 37 A 38 B

39. Multiplying factor for estimating stature from humerus is (males):

A. 10-12 **B.** 5-6
C. 7-9 **D.** 9-10

40. Eruption of temporary teeth will be completed by:

A. 1 to 1-1/2 years **B.** 2 to 2-1/2 years
C. 3 to 4 years **D.** 4 to 5 years

41. Foetal parts can be detected by X-ray usually by:

A. 8 weeks **B.** 12 weeks
C. 14 weeks **D.** 16 weeks

42. Union of epiphysis at the age of 17 occurs in:

A. Head of femur
B. Head of humerus
C. Lower end of femur
D. All of the above

43. A girl of 10 years will have ..... permanent and ..... temporary teeth.

A. 8, 12 **B.** 8, 16
C. 12, 12 **D.** 16, 8

44. Multiplying factor of estimating stature from femur (males) is:

A. 3.6-3.8 **B.** 4.1-4.8
C. 4.9-5.6 **D.** 5.8-6.2

45. The most reliable bones for the purpose of medullary index are the following *except:*

A. Humerus **B.** Tibia
C. Radius **D.** Sternum

46. Lower end of the femur can help to determine the:

A. Age **B.** Height
C. Weight **D.** Stature

---

39 B 40 B 41 D 42 A 43 D 44 A 45 D
46 A

47. The age of a 15-year-old female is best determined by the radiograph of:
A. Lower end of Radius and Ulna
B. Upper end of Humerus
C. Upper end of Radius and Ulna
D. Xiphisternum

48. Faint letter mark can be made visible by:
A. Infrared photography
B. Spectrophotometer
C. Ordinary light
D. X-rays

49. Which of the following is best for establishing identity?
A. Anthropometry
B. Dactylography
C. Hair examination
D. Blood

50. Human hair differs from animal hair by that:
A. Cuticle has scales
B. Medulla is thin
C. Medulla is broad than cortex
D. Pigment is central

51. A female pelvis differs from male pelvis by all *except:*
A. Obtuse subpubic angle
B. Broad greater sciatic foramen
C. Broad lesser sciatic foramen
D. Prominent muscle markings

52. Pearson's formula is used for:
A. Cephalic index **B.** Stature
C. Race **D.** Age

53. Closure of coronal sutures starts at the age of:
A. 20 years **B.** 21 years
C. 30-35 years **D.** 50-60 years

47 C 48 A 49 B 50 B 51 D 52 B 53 C

54. Pure Aryans have which type of skull?
A. Mesaticephalic
B. Bradycephalic
C. Dolicocephalic
D. None of the above

55. The hair examination is important for the following cases:
A. To find out its origin
B. To find the accused or victim
C. In cases of sexual assault
D. In cases of lead poisoning

56. A child at the age of 7 years has how many teeth?
A. 16 B. 20
C. 24 D. 28

57. In India, a boy below.......years cannot be charged with rape.
A. 12 B. 14
C. 21 D. No such limit

58. The minimum age for the appointment of Governor is:
A. 18 years B. 21 years
C. 35 years D. 45 years

59. Patella completely ossify by the age of:
A. 6 years B. 10 years
C. 14 years D. 21 years

60. Best specimen of bone for sex determination is:
A. Femur B. Pelvis
C. Skull D. Mandible

61. Best method to determine age upto 14 years is:
A. Ossification centres
B. Dentition
C. Anthropometry
D. Head circumference

---

54 C **55** A,B,C, D **56** C **57** D **58** C **59** C **60** B
61 B

62. Fragmentation of medulla of scalp hair is a feature of all *except*:
A. Negro race B. Mongolians
C. Caucasians D. Aryans

63. If angle of mandible is obtuse it means that the bone belongs to:
A. Adult male B. Adult female
C. Young female child D. Elderly person

64. Identical twins may not have:
A. Same DNA fingerprint
B. Same fingerprint pattern
C. Same blood group
D. Same HLA system

65. Edmund Locard is known for his:
A. System of personal identification using the body measurements
B. Fingerprint study
C. Formula for estimation of stature
D. Theory of exchange

66. Brachycephaly is due to fusion of:
A. Sagittal suture
B. Coronal suture
C. Parietal suture
D. Lambdoid suture

67. Best method for identification of human is:
A. Blood grouping
B. Dactylography
C. Anthropometry
D. Gustaffon's formula

68. 100% sure differentiation of sex is possible by pelvic assessment of:
A. Subpubic angle
B. Obturator foramen
C. Preauricular sulcus
D. Greater sciatic notch

62 A 63 C&D 64 B 65 D 66 B 67 B 68 D

69. Statutory rape is:

A. Rape of an insane woman
B. Rape of another person's wife
C. Rape in police custody
D. Rape of under 18 years

70. What is 'DNA' fingerprinting?

A. Identification of a person fingerprinting by using genetic enginering method
B. A record of a person's genetic make up
C. Identification of persons by genetic analysis
D. None of the above

71. Gustafson's method for age determination from teeth is useful in which one of the following age group?

A. Less than 5 years
B. 6-10 years
C. 11-15 years
D. Above 25 years

72. Absent fragmented medulla in hair is seen in:

A. Negroid
B. Aryans
C. Mongoloids
D. Caucasians

73. Consider the following statements:
DNA fingerprint is valuable in
1. Determination of blood group
2. Investigation of crime
3. Investigation of autoimmune disease
4. Determination of paternity
Of these statements:

A. 1 and 3 are correct
B. 3 and 4 are correct
C. 2 and 4 are correct
D. 1 and 2 are correct

74. Sexual consent cannot be given by a girl below:

A. 16 years
B. 17 years
C. 18 years
D. 21 years

69 D **70** C **71** D **72** C **73** C **74** C

75. First finger loop bureau was established in:

A. London B. Paris
C. Calcutta D. Madras

76. The period of mixed dentition is between the ages of:

A. 2-5 years B. 6-11 years
C. 12-14 years D. 15-17 years

77. 20 permanent teeth and 4* temporary teeth are seen at the age of:

A. 8 years B. 11 years
C. 9 years D. 12 years

78. When two objects come in contact, an exchange takes place. This is known as:

A. Galton exchange
B. Locard exchange principle
C. Chertillions system
D. Hasse rule

79. First permanent tooth to arise:

A. Incisor B. Canine
C. Premolar D. Molar

80. Cheiloscopy is the study of:

A. Foot prints B. Palatal prints
C. Fingerprints D. Lip prints

81. Cephalic index in Indians is:

A. 70-75 B. 75-80
C. 85-90 D. 90-95

82. Which one of the following permanent teeth are most erratic in eruption and of little value in determining age?

A. Third molars B. Premolars
C. Second molars D. Incisors

83. A person can give valid consent for routine physical examination if he is above the age of:

A. 12 years B. 14 years
C. 18 years D. 16 years

---

75 C 76 B 77 B 78 B 79 D 80 D 81 B
82 A 83 A

2

Thanatology–Taphonomy

Thanatos is Greek **God of death** (Indian God is *Yamaraaj*).

Thanatology deals with death in all its aspects.

Taphonomy* is an interdisciplinary applied scientific study of Postmortem Processes in Context, which include studying decomposition; transport of body; scavenging; and associated organisms (entomology).

Transplantation of Human Organ Act (1994): Sec 2(d) defines death as ***brainstem death.***

Sec 46 IPC: *The word "death" denotes the* death of a human being unless the contrary appears from the context.

Atria Mortis (Gateways of Death): Also known as **Modes of Death.**

Three modes of death are: (**Bichat**)

- Coma (Brain)
- Asphyxia (Lungs)
- Syncope (Heart).

Bishop's **"Tripod of life"** is Brain, Lungs and Heart.

Somatic Death: Clinically dead person with certain individual cells still functional.

Supra-Vital Interval: Period between somatic and cellular death. 1-2 hours*.

Cellular Death: All the cells of dead person cease to function.

Minnesota Criteria is for Brainstem Death (most modern* 1971).

Harvard Criteria (1968) and Philadelphia protocol are for Brain Death (1969).

Harvard Criteria of Brain Death

1. Unreceptivity and unresponsiveness.
2. No movements.
3. Apnoea: Absence of complete breathing for one hour.
4. Absence to elicit reflexes – Oculovestibular, Corneal, Pharyngeal **(Patellar Reflex or Deep Tendon Reflexes* may be present).**
5. Isoelectric EEG* Confirmatory test.

Rule of 'Two'

1. These criteria should be present for **TWO** hours.
2. **TWO** physicians should certify the death.

HOTTA–Human Organ and Tissue Transplantation Act

Step One – Proper Declaration of Brain Death

Any government certified transplant center or non-transplant organ retrieval center (NTORC) must have a **Brain Death Panel** in place.

This panel consists of 4 physicians:

1. The Registered Medical Practitioner (RMP) in charge of the hospital.
2. An independent RMP nominated by (1) above and approved by the State Appropriate Authority.
3. A Government appointed RMP; and
4. The RMP treating the patient.

(NB: The doctor who has to perform the transplant does not certify Brain Death, to avoid any conflict of interest or biased judgement**.)

It is the responsibility of the Brain Death Panel to perform the clinical brain death exam and confirmatory **Apnea test twice, at an interval of at least 6 hours.**

Responsibility of the Brain Death Panel

a. To explain to the patient's family the purpose and meaning of declaring brain death, completing the appropriate certifying documentation (**Form 10 is filled**).
b. To notify the hospital's Transplant Coordinator after the first brain death exam.
c. It should not be the responsibility of the Brain Death Panel to discuss organ donation with the family as this is the responsibility of the **Transplant Coordinator**.
   - In addition to human organs, HOTTA seeks to regulate transplantation of **tissues** of the human body.
   - The Act permits donations from living persons who are near relatives. The Bill expands the definition of "near relative" to include **grandparents and grandchildren** in addition to parents, children, brother, sister and spouse.
   - The doctor in an Intensive Care Unit **has to inform the patient** or relatives of patient about the option of organ donation and ascertain whether they would consent to the donation.
   - The Bill has made **punishment more severe**: Unauthorized removal–**5-10 years**/penalty up to Rs. 20 lakh.
     Commercial dealing–2-7 years/10,000-20,000.

- Donor >18 years.
- Organ harvesting from unclaimed bodies >48 hours.
- Bladder is not used from cadaver for organ transplantation.

Transplantation Period	
Lungs	: 15 minutes
Kidneys	: 45 minutes
Heart	: 1 hour
Cornea	: Preferable 2 hours (opacities)–max 6 hours
Skin	: 24 hours
Bone	: 48 hours
Blood Vessels	: 72 hours

Euthanasia–the idea of a good death.

A. Direct Euthanasia

- o *Passive Euthanasia*, which lets a sick person die.
- o *Active Euthanasia*, a second person who helps the patient to die.
- o Supreme Court of India has allowed **passive euthanasia under "exceptional circumstances"**, it has made clear that active euthanasia is illegal.

B. Indirect Euthanasia (also known as double effect): An act of providing the patient with treatment to alleviate his or her suffering resulting in the death of the patient.

C. Cacotanasia: The practice of euthanasia without the consent of the patient.

D. Ortotanasia, when a terminally ill patient is allowed to die once their time has come.

E. Dysthanasia: The idea of a **bad death**. Every possible method is used to prolong the life of a terminally ill person.

- Declaration of Sydney – Definition of Death.
- Declaration of Venice – Terminal Illness.

Named Tests for Detection of Breathing and Circulation

Signs of Death:

Circulation:

1. **Diaphanus test:** Finger webs lose lusture, a circulation test.
2. **I card's dye test:** Dye injected I.V., colour does not change in dead. It is a test for circulation.
3. **Magnus test:** Ligature applied to finger. It swells and becomes blue if the person is alive, test for circulation.

Respiration:

4. **Winslow's test:** Reflections from mirror over chest move with **respirations*** if alive.

POSTMORTEM CHANGES

Signs of Death and Changes Following Death

Signs of death appear in the following order:

1. **Immediate** (somatic death):
   a. Insensibility and loss of voluntary power* → earliest sign at death.
   b. Cessation of respiration.
   c. Cessation of circulation.
2. **Early** (cellular death):
   a. Pallor and loss of elasticity of skin.
   b. Changes in the eye.
   c. Primary flaccidity of muscles.
   d. Cooling of the body.
   e. Postmortem lividity.
   f. Rigor mortis.
3. **Late** (decomposition and decay):
   a. Putrefaction.
   b. Adipocere formation.
   c. Mummification.

Suspended Animation (Apparent Death, Death Trance)

- In this condition, **no signs of life are discovered** as the functions are interrupted for some time or are reduced to minimum.
- However, **life continues** and resuscitation is successful in such cases.
- Voluntarily, practitioners of yoga can pass into a trance, death-like in character.
- Involuntary suspension of animation lasting from a few seconds to half-an-hour may be found in:
  - A—After Anesthesia
  - **B—in newborn infants**
  - C—Cholera/Cerebral concussion
  - D—Drowning
  - **E—Electrocution**
  - Shock, Sunstroke, inSanity, etc.

Changes in Eye

- **Rail roading phenomenon:** Fragmentation or segmentation (trucking) of the blood columns in the retinal vessels appear **within minutes** after death. This is also known as '**Kevorkian Sign**'.
- Cornea becomes opaque in 2 to 4 hours (Corneal cloudiness develops within 3 hours of death).
- Intra-ocular tension falls after death.

Living Humans = 15-25 gms
Soon after death = 3-12 gms
After 30 mins = less than 3 gms
(*3-zero-3 gms.* memory cue)
After 2 hours = Zero.

- **Taches noires de Sclerotica** appear within **3 hours** of death on *sclera.** Cell debris and mucus forms yellow triangle on each side of cornea.
- Potassium level steadily **rise*** in vitreous [**K**rishh! Ri-eyes (**rise**)].

Cooling of the Body (Algor Mortis)

- Internal organs take 24 hours to cool.
- Most useful single indicator for postmortem interval during the first 24 hours after death.
- The curve of cooling is **sigmoid or inverted (mirror image of) 'S' in pattern.** **The Henssge nomogram (HN) is used for calculating time of death based on body temperature measurement(s).**

HN Relies Upon

1. The body weight.
2. The environmental temperature; and
3. The measured deep rectal temperature with assumption that a normal body temperature at death of 37.2 C.
   [N.B.→ Ordinary clinical thermometer is useless, hence a chemical thermometer, which is 25–30 cm long with a range from 0 to 50 C is ideally used].

Alternative site for Core Temperature–**Subhepatic.**

- A rough idea of time in hours of death can be obtained by:

$$\frac{\textit{(Normal body temperature–Rectal temperature)}}{\textit{Rate of temperature fall per hour}}$$

- A rule of thumb to estimate time since death is:

$$\frac{\textit{Normal:}\text{ Body temperature—Rectal temperature (Temperature in °F)}}{1.5}$$

or (Normal Body Temperature—Rectal temp) × 0.67 (°**F**) (N.B.T.—R.T.) × 2 (°**C**)
Rate of fall of temperature is—1.5 (°**F**)/Hr or 0.5 (°**C**)/Hr

Classical 'rules of thumb'
• Body temperature falls by 1.5°F (<1°C) per hour • Time since death (in hours) = fall in body temperature from 37°C + 3 (**why +3 ?**: First 3 hours after death body shows "postmortem temperature plateau/ isothermic phase") • Skin feels cold 2-4 hours postmortem indoors (6-8 hours in protected areas)

- Low temperature occurs in cases of:
  - Collapse
  - Congestive cardiac failure
  - Massive hemorrhage etc.

Postmortem Caloricity*

The temperature of the body remains high for the first two hours.

Conditions resulting in postmortem caloricity:

i. Disturbance of heat regulation
   - Sunstroke
   - Pontine hemorrhage.

ii. Increased production of heat due to muscular activity
   - Tetanus
   - Strychnin, Heroin, Cocaine.

iii. Excessive bacterial activity
- Septicemia
- Cholera.

LIVOR MORTIS (Postmortem Staining)

- **Synonyms** of postmortem staining are cadaveric lividity, hypostasis, ***suggilations****, vibices* or livor mortis.
- Cadaveric lividity is an **early** sign of death.
- Postmortem hypostasis is bluish purple or purplish red discoloration, which appears under the skin (rete mucosum) of the dependent part of the body after death due to **capillovenous distention*.**
- Postmortem lividity begins shortly after death, but it may not be visible for about half to one hour after death.
- It is usually well developed **within 4 hours** and reaches a maximum **between 6 and 12 hours**.
- The postmortem staining gets fixed in **6-7 hours**.
- Postmortem hypostasis persists till it merges with discoloration of putrefaction.
- It is more marked in asphyxia and is less marked in death from hemorrhage, anemia, lobar pneumonia and wasting disease.

Location of Postmortem Hypostasis

- ***In case of Hanging:*** Hypostasis is more marked in lower limbs, external genitals, lower part of arms and forearms.
- ***In case of Drowning:*** If the body is constantly moving, P.M. staining may not develop.
- In a body lying on its back, it first appears in the neck and then spreads over the entire back except parts directly pressed on, i.e., shoulder-blades, buttocks, calves and heel.
- Postmortem staining can occur in some cases before death in **cholera**.
- As decomposition progresses, the lividity becomes dusky in colour and turns brown and green before finally disappearing with destruction of the blood.

- The hypostatic areas have a distinct colour in certain cases of poisoning, e.g.,
  1. In carbon monoxide poisoning–**cherry red.**
  2. In hydrocyanic and poisoning–**bright red.**
  3. In poisoning by nitrites, potassium chlorate, nitrobenzene, aniline (causing methaemoglobinaemia) the colour is **red brown or brown.**
  4. In potassium cyanide poisoning–**Deep blue.**
  5. In clostridum perfringens infection–**Bronze** colour.
  6. Bright pink–**Hypothermia.**
  7. Black colour—**Opium*.**
  8. **H2S poisoning–Bluish Green.**
- **Medicolegal Importance**
  1. It indicates posture of body at the time of death.
  2. Colour indicates cause of death.
  3. Postmortem lividity in comparison to bruise has characteristics:
     a. Epidermal in situation
     b. Seen in dependent part
     c. Uniform in colour.
  4. Antemortem clot is firm, does not wash out, brown in colour, but postmortem clot is **friable.**
  5. Congestion of organs can be mistaken for hypostasis.

Muscular Changes

- After death, the muscles of the body pass through **three stages:**
  1. Primary relaxation or flaccidity.
  2. Rigor mortis.
  3. Secondary flaccidity.

1. **Primary Flaccidity**
   - During the stage, death is only somatic, and it lasts for one to three hours.
2. **Rigor Mortis (Sommer's Movements is seen due to R.M.)**

Definition

- This is stage of **stiffening of muscles with shortening** of the fibers.
- Individual cell death takes place at this stage.
- It develops 3 hours after death.

Mechanism

- When the ATP is **reduced** to **85%** of the normal, the overlapping portions of myosin and action filaments combine as rigid links of actomyosin, which is viscous and inextensible and causes hardness and rigidity of muscle rigor.
- When lactic acid concentration reaches a level of **0.5%,** muscles go into rigor mortis (pH level fall).
- Rigor persists until decomposition of the proteins of the muscle fibers makes them incapable of any further contraction.

The Order of Appearance of Rigor Mortis

- All muscles of the body, both voluntary and involuntary are affected.
- It first appears in **involuntary muscles**–the **myocardium** becomes rigid in **an hour.**
- Involuntary muscle in:
  - Order of **onset of** rigor mortis is–**eyelids**–thorax–lower limbs.
  - Order of **disappearance** of rigor mortis is–**eyelids**–thorax–lower extremities.
- *Nysten's Law** deals with **progression of Rigor** in different muscles.
- When rigor is fully developed, the entire body is **stiff,** the muscles shortened, hard and opaque.

Time of Onset

- In **India,** it begins **1 to 2 hours** after death and takes further 1 to 2 hours to develop.
- In temperate countries, it begins in 3 to 6 hours and takes further 2 to 3 hours to develop.

Duration of Rigor Mortis

- Rigor mortis follows ***"RULE OF 12"***→12 hours to set in, 12 hours to remain, 12 hours to pass off. It takes roughly 36 hours for rigor mortis to vanish.

Conditions Altering the Onset and Duration

General Rule: Onset of rigor is accelerated and its duration shortened when the environmental temperature is high and after prolonged muscular activity for e.g.:

- In death from diseases causing great exhaustion and wasting, e.g., cholera, typhoid, tuberculosis, cancer, etc. and in violent death as cut-throat, firearm, electrocution, heat stroke, strychnine poisoning.

Medicolegal Importance

- The rigor mortis sets faster in children, elderly, malnourished individuals; body immersed in water.
- Causes delaying the onset of rigor mortis are– pneumonia, apoplexy, myasthenia gravis.

Conditions Simulating Rigor Mortis

1. **Heat Stiffening**
   - When body is exposed to temperature above 60°C, rigidity is produced.
   - It is seen in deaths from burning, high voltage electric shock, from falling into hot liquids.
   - **Pugilistic Attitude** is seen due to coagulation of proteins in both Antemortem and Postmortem *Burns**.
2. **Cold Stiffening**
   - When the body is exposed to freezing temperatures, the tissues become frozen and stiff.
3. **Cadaveric Spasm or Instantaneous Rigor or Cataleptic Rigidity***
   - In this condition, the muscles that are

contracted during life, become stiff and rigid immediately after death, **without the stage of primary relaxation**.

- It occurs especially in cases of:

  A–sudden **A**sphyxial death

  B–injury to the **B**rain

  C–**C**erebral hemorrhage

  D–**D**rowning, *Di–nitro–Ortho Cresol* poisoning

  E–**E**xhaustion

  F–**F**ear, **F**irearm injury.

- This is usually limited to a **single group of muscles** and frequently involves hands.
- It mainly occurs in **voluntary muscles.**
- It cannot be produced by any method after death.
- It may be explained on the basis of diminished or exhausted ATP in the affected muscles.
- Rigor mortis **simulates cadaveric spasm.**

Difference Between Rigor Mortis and Cadaveric Spasm:

	Trait	*Rigor mortis*	*Cadaveric spasm*
1.	Production	Freezing and exposure to temperature above 65°C will produce rigor	Cannot be produced artificially
2.	Mechanism	Known	Not clearly known
3.	Predisposing	Nil	Sudden death, excitement, fear, exhaustion, nervous tension, etc.
4.	Time of onset	One to two hours after death	Instantaneous
5.	Muscles involved	All the muscles of the body, both voluntary and involuntary	Usually limited to a **single group of voluntary** muscles
6.	Muscle stiffening	Not marked	Marked
7.	Molecular death	Occurs	Does not occur
8.	Body heat	Cold	Warm
9.	Electrical stimuli	Muscles do not respond	Muscles respond
10.	Medicolegal importance	Indicates **time of** death	Indicates **modes of** death, i.e., suicide, homicide or accident

Medicolegal Importance

- In case of suicide, the weapon, e.g., pistol or knife is seen firmly grasped in victim's hand which is a strong presumptive evidence of suicide.

- In cases of drowning, material such as grass, weeds etc. may be found firmly grasped in the hand, which shows **antemortem drowning.**

4. **Embalming**
   - The contents of the body cavities are removed, and the vascular system is injected with an embalming fluid.
   - Typically embalming fluid contains a **mixture of formaldehyde (NOT formalin*), methanol, ethanol, phenol, glycerin and other solvents.** The formaldehyde content generally ranges from 5 to 29 percent and the ethanol content may range from 9 to 56 percent.
   - Formalin refers specifically to 37% aqueous formaldehyde and is not commonly used in funeral embalming but **rather in the preservation of anatomical specimens**.
   - **Purpose:** Slow the decomposition of the body.
   - **Embalming is never done before postmortem*** because it alters the appearance of the body, tissues and organs, making it difficult to interpret any injury or disease. Embalming completely destroys cyanide, alcohol and many other substances. Determination of the presence of many of the alkaloids and organic poisons becomes very difficult.
   - **The viscera** should be refrigerated at about **4°C,** if not forwarded to the chemical examiner. They can be destroyed either after getting the permission from the Magistrate, or when the investigating police officer informs that the case has been closed.
   - Body should not be undressed before the forensic doctor has seen it as it may suppress significant information.
   - For longer duration, viscera can be stored at –20°C.

Secondary Relaxation

- Muscles become soft and flaccid due to breaking down of actomyosin due to putrefaction.

Putrefaction

- Putrefaction is the final stage following death, produced mainly by the action of bacterial enzymes, mostly anaerobic organism derived from the bowel.
- Enzymes **Lecithinase** produced by **Cl. Welchii** is most important.
- The **characteristic features** of putrefaction are:
  - Changes in the colour of the tissue.
  - Collection of gases in the tissues.
  - Liquefaction of tissues.
- The **first external sign of putrefaction**
  - In a body lying in air is a greenish discoloration of skin over caecum, i.e., **right iliac fossa.***
  - **Sulphmeth haemoglobin** causes greenish discoloration.*
  - The **color appears** in 12 to 18 hours in summer and 1 to 2 days in winter.
- The **earliest internal change** is reddish brown discoloration of the **inner surface of the vessels,** especially the aorta.
- The **marbled** appearance is prominent **in 36 to 48 hours.**
- Due to the presence of gases in the abdomen, the diaphragm is forced upwards resulting in expulsion of blood stained froth/gastric contents from mouth and nostrils—POSTMORTEM PURGE.*
- After 3 days, the face is so discolored and bloated that identification becomes difficult. The hair becomes loose and is easily pulled out.

Putrefaction Crystals: Yellowish particles composed of tyrosine and leucine, found on the surface and bottom side of the liver.

The **liver** shows spongy consistency, in more advanced stages of putrefaction gives a **Swiss-Cheese-like appearance.**

Postmortem Luminescence

It is caused by contamination by:

1. Armillaria Mellea/Ramsbottom (fungi).
2. **Photobacterium fischeri** (bacteria).
   - **Colliquative putrefaction** begins from 5 to 10 days after death.
   - The organs show **putrefactive changes** in the following order:
     1. Larynx and trachea
     2. Stomach, intestines, spleen
     3. Liver and lungs
     4. Brain
     5. Uterus, prostate
     6. Skin, muscle tendon
     7. Bone.
   - In putrefaction, liver has a **honey combed** or **foamy appearance.**
   - **Prostate and non-gravid uterus** resist putrefaction for a very long time.
   - Putrefaction begins above 10°C and optimum between 21°C and 38°C.
   - ***Casper's Dictum**** "A body decomposes in air ***twice*** as rapidly as in water ***and eight times*** as rapidly as in earth".

     [1 week of putrefaction in air is equivalent to 2 weeks in water, which is equivalent to 8 weeks buried in soil].

     Putrefaction is rapid when body is buried in:
     - Damp
     - Marshy
     - Shallow graves.
   - Putrefaction is **surest sign of death.**
   - Antibiotics before death slows down putrefaction.
   - Nuclear features persist in decomposition for a period of 2-3 years.
   - Bones begin to decompose after death in 3-10 years.

- Less than 7 amino acids in bone suggest the age of bone to be (after death) more than 100 years.
- **First amino acid** to disappear is **Proline and Hydroxy-Proline.***
- Last amino acid to disappear is **Glycine.***
- Total ultraviolet fluorescence of cut surface of bones is seen in 35-100 years.

Pink Teeth Phenomenon

Pink coloration of teeth may occur some time after death under conditions that promote putrefaction and adipocere formation. The red coloration is due to hemolysis after exudation of hemoglobin derivatives through the dentine tubules in cases in which blood has accumulated in the head, either due to congestion or by a postmortem head-down position, as after submersion in water. It is also a common finding related to cases of asphyxia such as strangulation, drowning or suffocation.

Maceration

- Sterile autolysis of an unborn fetus–died in utero enclosed within the amniotic cavity.
- The most prominent finding is skin slippage with underlying brownish-blackish discoloration of tissue.
- **M/L Importance:** The presence of maceration without any putrefactive changes in a recently delivered child is indicative of **stillbirth**.

Potential Question Zone

Putrefaction vs. Autolysis

Autolysis differs from Putrefaction as it is a pure result of endogenous enzyme activity and bacterial processes play no role. The earliest sign of **autolysis** is a whitish, cloudy appearance of the cornea.

Putrefaction vs. Decomposition

Decomposition is the product of soft-tissue degradation by **Aerobic bacteria**, originating from outside environmental sources. Putrefaction is the bacterial degradation of soft tissue by **Anaerobic bacteria,** e.g., Clostridium, Proteus species, originating from the gut into blood vessels and into tissue and then to the whole body.

Changes in Vitreous Humor

K^+ level rises in linear fashion with increase in time since death.

Formulas used to calculate K^+ level are:

- **Sturner's Formula.**
- **Madea's Formula.**

Entomology of cadaver is the study of insects and maggots that infest the dead body. Maggots in a dead body do not appear **before 48 hours.**

- **Megnin*** studied ***the 8 waves*** of infestation of body by different species of insects.

Methods of Estimation of Time Since Death in Forensic Archeology

- Estimation of radioactive carbon (half life = 5,600 years).
- **Flow cytometry:** Method of estimation of **degree of degradation of DNA** compared to those whose time of death is known.

Adipocere (Saponification, Corpse Wax)

Sir Thomas Browne discovered adipocere.

1. It is seen in body immersed in water or damp warm environment.
   Cold temp (4-7d) and Hot temp (decompose) are unfavorable for adipocere formation {Optimal Temp is required}.

Favourable for adipocere	*Unfavourable for adipocere*
1. Fat, female, newborn	1. Thin, male, older
2. Room temperature (36 hrs)	2. Cold temp (4-7d): Hot temp (decompose) [MCQ*]
3. Autumn or winter	3. Spring and summer
4. Fog, misty and humid	4. Dry
5. More deep graves	5. Shallow or surface graves
6. Oak, lead n Zn coffins	6. Pine n sprue coffins
7. *pH >7**	

2. Adipocere contains:
   - Palmitic acid.
   - Oleic acid.
   - Hydroxy-stearic acid.
   - Stearic acid.
3. The **change** is due to gradual *hydrolysis and hydrogenation* of pre-existing fat. Water for hydrolysis is obtained from body tissues.
4. Intrinsic lipases and clostridium, perfringens are responsible for adipocere formation.
5. Adipocere is **delayed** by cold and **formed rapidly** by warm humid climate.
6. It has ammoniacal odour.
7. **Fresh adipocere** is soft, moist, whitish and translucent resembles **RANCID BUTTER*** but old samples are dry, hard, cracked, yellowish and brittle.
8. It is formed first in **subcutaneous tissue.**
   - In temperate country, the shortest time for its **formation** is about 3 weeks in summer.
   - In India, it has been observed within 3 days.
   - Fetus under 7 months do not show this change.
   - The presence of oxygen inhibits adipocere formation.

Mummification

- It is **modification of putrefaction,** occur when the environmental condition is hot and dry.
- Mummification occurs when body is buried in dry sandy shallow graves.*

- **Desiccation*** **or** dehydration or drying and shrinkage of the cadaver occur due to evaporation of water but the natural appearance and features of the body are preserved.
- A mummified body is **odourless.**
- The **time required for complete mummification of a body** varies from three months to a year or two.
- Arsenic and antimony poisoning favors it.

Types of Mummification

i. **Primary Mummification** is generally NOT accompanied by putrefaction, occur in environment that favor a rapid drying of soft tissues.
ii. **Secondary Mummification** follows considerable putrefaction of the body. Secondary mummification is seen more often in open spaces than indoors.

Exhumation (Origin: Ex-out Humus-Soil)

- Exhumation is the digging out of an already buried body from the grave.
- There is no time limit for exhumation in India.
- The body is exhumed only when there is a written order from the **first class magistrate (Chief Judicial Magistrate) or first class executive magistrate (DM).**
- Police cannot order Exhumation.
- It should be conducted in natural light in early morning.
- Average number of sample of earth taken is 6-7.
- Disinfectants should not be sprinkled on the body.
- In suspected mineral poisoning, hair, nails and long bone, e.g., femur should be preserved for chemical analysis.
- It is not done for Hindus, performed for Christians, Muslims and Parsies.

Presumption of Survivorship

(S→seven/survivorship)

Sec 107 IEA→Burden of proving death of a person known to have been alive and age within **30 years.**

Presumption of Death

Sec 108 IEA→Burden of proving a person is alive unheard of for **7 years**.

MEDICOLEGAL AUTOPSY

(Also known as Obduction, Necropy, Thanatopsy)

Literal Meaning – "To see for oneself").

Bartolomeo da Varignana performed the first medicolegal autopsy in **Bologna, Italy.**

Temperature (Algor M) × Rigidity (Rigor M) Matrix (Time since Death)		
	Not Rigid	**Rigid**
Warm	Not more than 3 hours	3-8 hours
Cold	More than 36 hours	8-36 hours

Sequence of Opening Body Cavities at Autopsy

A. If cause of death is not apparent the following order of organ examination must be followed:

1. Heart (Opened in direction of blood flow Rt. Atrium→Rt. Ventricle→Lt. Atrium→Lt. Ventricle using an instrument **ENTERO-TOME***).
2. Pulmonary arteries.
3. Brain–externally and with one cut to the pons.
4. Larynx and trachea.
5. Remainder of organs.

B. Asphyxia – Cranium is opened first. Neck is opened last.

C. Poisoning–Cranium is opened first. Abdomen last.
D. Head Injury–Cranium opened first.
(Cranium is opened first as a general rule).

Types of Incisions:

- **I Shaped**–Most common.
- **Y Shaped**–Neck Trauma, Mechanical Asphyxia.
- **Inverted Y Shaped**–Upto umbilicus I shaped and then 2 limbs of incision towards both flanks. **Fetus and Newborns.**

AUTOPSY TECHNIQUES

Virchow Technique

- Organs are removed one by one and dissected as removed.
- Most widely used method with some modifications.
- Good for demonstrating pathological change in individual organs, especially in high risk autopsies.

Disadvantage: Relationships between various organs may be hard to interpret.

Rokitansky Technique

Partial *in situ* dissection with en bloc removal. **Infected Corpse, Children.**

Technique of M. Letulle

Thoracic, cervical, abdominal and pelvic organs are removed *en masse* and subsequently dissected into organ blocks. Best technique for preserving the vascular supply and relationships between organs.

Technique of Gohn

Organ systems are removed separately as organ blocks.

Compromise between **Letulle and Virchow technique.**

Pediatric Autopsies

- Follows the technique described by Potter and Craig*.
- Langley technique for perinatal autopsies.
- Skull is opened using
  a. Beneke technique – two flaps
  b. Barr's Technique: Opened in 4 flaps (Butterfly Formation).
- In most instances the Letulle technique is used.

Autopsy of Spinal Cord

- **Three approaches used to open:** Anterior, Posterior and Anterolateral.
- **Most commonly used approach:** Anterior.
- **BEST approach to examine spinal cord: Posterior.**

Posterior vs. Anterior

Posterior Approach: This method allows easy exposure of the uppermost cervical spine and allows direct visualization of the craniocervical junction; it is therefore recommended in **(COMA).**

- **C**raniocervical instability.
- **O**ccipital encephalocele.
- **M**yelomeningocele.
- **A**rnold-Chiari malformation.

Most morticians **object to the routine use of this method**, because embalming fluids tend to leak from the incision on the back. It is **much less suited** for pursuing the course of peripheral nerves for any length in contiguity with the spinal cord.

Anterior Approach: The anterior approach is simple and quick and does not require turning the body over. It also permits removal of the spinal cord and peripheral nerves in continuity when indicated. Immediate examination of the vertebral bodies is an **added advantage.**

TYPES OF ARTEFACTS

1. Due to resuscitative or therapeutic measures.
2. Between Death and Autopsy (Agonal Artefacts). Any change or feature introduced into the body after death that is likely to lead to misinterpretation of medicolegally significant antemortem findings. The autopsy pathologist should be able to distinguish them from significant antemortem changes.
3. Due to injuries or lesions of organs before death.
4. During autopsy.

False Simulated Artificial Bruise

- Irritant substances like Plumbago Zeylanica, Rolsea, Semicarpus Anacardium.
- Margins contain tiny vesicles containing acrid serous fluid.
- Diagnosis is made by **incision, clot cannot be wiped off.**
- Done to substantiate a false charge of assault.

Kennedy's Phenomenon: Artefacts in respect to gun-shot wounds. Surgical/Medical intervention – cleaning debridement etc., removes gun powder, and changes the over all character gun-shot wounds as in J.F. Kennedy murder case.

Prinsloo and Gordon Artefact: Artefactual extravasation of blood into the anterior neck structures at autopsy, resembling traumatic bruises. A layered *in-situ* approach to the neck dissection, prevents this artefact.

MCQs

1. **Time limit for exhumation in India is:**
   A. 10 years B. 20 years
   C. 30 years D. No time limit
2. **Suspended animation may be found in following conditions *except:***
   A. Drowning B. Electrocution
   C. Throttling D. Hypothermia
3. **Intraocular tension is nil after death in about:**
   A. 1 hour B. 2 hours
   C. 3 hours D. 4 hours
4. **Postmortem caloricity is seen in poisoning from:**
   A. Cyanide B. Opium
   C. Arsenic D. Strychnine
5. **Fixation of hypostasis occur in about:**
   A. 2 hours B. 4 hours
   C. 6 hours D. 12 hours
6. **Patchy postmortem hypostasis can be seen:**
   A. Immediately after death
   B. Half hours to one after death
   C. 2-3 hours after death
   D. 4-6 hours after death
7. **Length of oesophagus in adults is about:**
   A. 18 cm B. 22 cm
   C. 25 cm D. 30 cm
8. **First structure to show rigor mortis is:**
   A. Eye lids B. Lips
   C. Heart D. Intestines

1 D 2 C 3 B 4 D 5 C 6 B

7 C 8 C

9. Rigor mortis only develop in a foetus after the age of:

A. 3 months **B.** 5 months
C. 7 months **D.** 9 months

10. First external sign of putrefaction is:

A. Greenish discoloration of abdomen
B. Distension of abdomen
C. Marbling of skin
D. Protrusion of tongue

11. Rate of putrefaction of a dead body in air than buried in soil:

A. Same **B.** Twice
C. Four times **D.** Eight times

12. Bacteria helpful in *adipocere* formation is:

A. B proteus
B. B coli
C. Slaphylococci
D. Cl Welchii

13. Rate of growth of beard hair is:

A. 0.2 mm/day **B.** 0.4 mm/day
C. 0.6 mm/day **D.** 1 mm/day

14. Last organ to purify in human body is:

A. Heart **B.** Kidneys
C. Prostate **D.** Ovaries

15. *Tachae noires* are seen after death in the eyes in about:

A. 3 hours **B.** 6 hours
C. 12 hours **D.** 18 hours

16. In pugilistic attitude which of the following statement is correct?

A. It is antemortem in nature
B. ATP depletion is the cause
C. Generalised extension of the body present
D. Coagulation of muscle proteins is present

---

9 C **10 A** **11 D** **12 D** **13 B** **14 C**

15 A **16 D**

17. In myocardial infraction microscopic changes cannot be observed before:

A. 4 hours B. 8 hours
C. 12 hours D. 16 hours

18. In maceration which of the following statement is not true?

A. A sterile condition
B. Foetus is flaccid
C. Emits sweetish but disagreeable smell
D. Skin assumes greenish colour

19. Preservative used routinely for preserving viscera for chemical analysis is:

A. 10% formaline
B. Saturated common salt solution
C. Rectified spirit
D. Normal saline

20. Immediate rigidity of a group of muscles is called:

A. Cadaveric rigidity
B. Cadaveric rigidity
C. Cataleptic rigidity
D. Algar mortis

21. Rigor mortis develops..............after death.

A. 1/2-1 hour B. 1 to 2 hours
C. 3 to 6 hours D. 6 to 8 hours
E. 12 hours

22. Cadaveric spasm:

A. Instant in onset
B. Confined to a small group of muscle
C. Occurs only in voluntary muscles
D. Indicates that the person was alive at that time
E. All of the above

23. Foamy liver is seen in:

A. Putrefaction B. Drowning
C. Mummification D. Adipocere

---

17 B 18 D 19 B 20 C 21 C 22 E
23 A

24. Postmortem staining gets fixed after:

A. 2-3 hours
B. 3-4 hours
C. 5-6 hours
D. 6-7 hours
E. 7-8 hours

25. Mummification occurs when:

A. High atmospheric temperature is present
B. Dry air condition
C. Wind is present
D. All are correct

26. If a body is left undisturbed for how long does postmortem staining persists?

A. Few hours
B. Few days
C. Few months
D. Persists till it merges with discolouration of putrefaction

27. Suspended animation may be seen in:

A. Electrocution
B. Morphine poisoning
C. Strangulation
D. Rape

28. Hypostasis lasts for:

A. Hours
B. Days
C. Weeks
D. Months

29. Cadaveric spasm:

A. Immediately after death
B. After 2 hours of death
C. Affect voluntary muscles
D. Affects involuntary muscle

30. The rate of cooling down of dead bodies in tropical climate is:

A. 0.2°C/hour
B. 0.5°C/hour
C. 1.0°C/hour
D. 1.5°C/hour

31. Last organ to be affected in putrefaction:

A. Prostate
B. Uterus
C. Kidney
D. Thyroid

---

24 D 25 D 26 D 27 A 28 B 29 A,C
30 B 31 A, B

32. Immediate stiffness postmortem occurs in:
A. Cadaveric rigidity
B. Cadaveric spasm
C. Rigor mortis
D. Algor mortis

33. Ossification centre appearing just before birth is:
A. Lower end of femur
B. Lower end of tibia
C. Upper end of humerus
D. Scaphoid

34. Mummification is:
A. Desiccation of the body
B. Pugilistic attitude of the body
C. Electric burns
D. Burking

35. The most common cause for sudden death is:
A. Acute myocarditis
B. Pulmonary edema
C. Myocardial infarction
D. CCF

36. Floatation of a body in water is due to:
A. Flesh being eaten by fishes
B. Presence of gases
C. Waterlogging of body
D. All of the above

37. Honeycombing is seen in liver in cases of:
A. Cirrhosis
B. Rupture
C. Putrefaction
D. Hydatid disease

38. Medicolegal autopsy requires the permission of:
A. Police
B. Magistrate
C. Relatives
D. Medical Superintendent

32 B 33 A 34 A 35 C 36 B 37 C
38 A

39. Presence of maggots at postmortem indicates:

A. Duration since death
B. Cause of death
C. Mode of death
D. Posture of body at time of death

40. Rigor mortis simulated by:

A. Mummification
B. Algor mortis
C. Cadaveric spasm
D. All of the above

41. Postmortem lividity is unlikely to develop in a case of:

A. Drowning in well
B. Drowning in a fast flowing river
C. Postmortem submersion
D. Drowning of chlorinated swimming pool

42. Cold stiffening may be associated with:

A. Trench foot
B. Immersion foot
C. Body rigid, heavy and stiff
D. Any of the above

43. Colour changes of putrefaction are first observed in the:

A. Iliac fossae
B. Popliteal fossae
C. Cubital fossae
D. Arm pits
E. Neck

44. Rigor mortis in India in summers sets in:

A. 2-3 hours
B. 18-36 hours
C. 2-5 days
D. 1 week

45. Numbers of hours since death is calculated by multiplying the fall in rectal temperature with:

A. 0.33
B. 0.67
C. 1.0
D. 1.33
E. 1.5

---

39 A **40 C** **41 B** **42 C** **43 A** **44 A**

45 B

46. Definition of suspended animation is:

A. It is a condition of apparent death when no signs of life are discovered as the functions are interrupted for some time or are reduced to minimum

B. Signs of death are irreversible

C. Only signs of brain death are present

D. None of the above

47. Colliquative liquefaction is seen within .... after death.

A. Immediately **B.** 24 hours

C. 72 hours **D.** 1 week

48. In putrefaction greenish discolouration is first seen in:

A. Loin **B.** Epigastrium

C. Right iliac fossa **D.** Lower limb

49. Maggots in a dead body do not appear before:

A. 4 hours **B.** 12 hours

C. 24 hours **D.** 48 hours

50. The temperature of the body rises up for the first two hours after death. The probable condition include following *except*:

A. Sun-stroke **B.** Frost-bite

C. Septicemia **D.** Tetanus

E. Strychnine poisoning

51. Postmortem staining can occur in some cases before death in:

A. Children **B.** Old persons

C. Cholera **D.** All of the above

52. The following are correct about cadaveric rigidity in contract to cadaveric spasm *except:*

A. Condition is seen after death

B. Affects in all muscles of body

C. Helpful in determining time since death

D. None of the above

---

46 A **47 D** **48 C** **49 D** **50 B** **51 C**

52 D

53. Rigor mortis first starts in:
A. Upper eyelids
B. Lower eyelids
C. Lower limbs
D. Fingers

54. "Cardiac polyp" is a term used for postmortem:
A. Fibrinous clots in heart
B. Aneurysm
C. Infarcts in heart
D. Pale patches in heart

55. Marbling is noticed by:
A. 18 hours
B. 36 hours
C. 48 hours
D. 24 hours

56. In rigor mortis muscle:
A. Stiffens
B. Shortens
C. Stiffens and shortens
D. Stiffens and lengthens

57. Putrefaction is a:
A. Perimortem sign of death
B. Immediate sign of death
C. Early sign of death
D. Late sign of death

58. Adipocere is likely to occur in:
A. Warm humid climate
B. Dry hot climate
C. Burial in sandy soil
D. All the above

59. Postmortem caloricity is seen with:
A. Strychnine poisoning
B. Lead poisoning
C. Mercury poisoning
D. Phosphorus poisoning

---

53 A **54 A** **55 B** **56 C** **57 D** **58 A**
59 A

60. First indication of postmortem putrefaction is:

A. Discolouration of right iliac fossa
B. Puffiness of face
C. Bullous lesion
D. Scaling of skin

61. Immediate rigidity of a group of muscle without passing into stage of primary relaxation:

A. Cadaveric spasm
B. Cadaveric rigidity
C. None of the above
D. All of the above

62. Maggots are seen on the dead body after:

A. One day **B.** 2 to 3 days
C. 3-4 days **D.** One week

63. The following situations are associated with rise of temperature after death *except:*

A. Burns
B. Heat stroke
C. Pontine haemorrhage
D. Septicaemia

64. Rate of cooling helps in determining:

A. Time of death
B. Manner of death
C. Place of death
D. Cause of death

65. Maggots appear in body in rainy season within:

A. 24 hours **B.** 1-2 days
C. 2-3 days **D.** 3-4 days

66. What is suspended animation?

A. Animal is suspended in air
B. The subject is alive but shows no signs of life
C. Hibernation
D. Deep sleep

---

60 A 61 A 62 B 63 A 64 A 65 B
66 B

67. Suspended animation occurs after:
A. Electrocution
B. Cyanide poisoning
C. Burns
D. Drowning

68. Putrefaction starts in:
A. Liver
B. Lung
C. Brain
D. Heart

69. Rigor mortis first starts in:
A. Heart
B. Eyelids
C. Lung
D. Limbs

70. Stellate wound is produced with firearm in:
A. Contact shot
B. Close shot
C. Range within 60 cms
D. Distant shot

71. Rigor mortis occurs first in which voluntary muscle?
A. Muscles of eyelids
B. Small muscles of hands
C. Neck muscles
D. Face muscles

72. Entomology of cadaver helps in finding:
A. Time since death
B. Mode of death
C. Manner of death
D. Identify the deceased

73. Temperature of a dead person is best measured by:
A. Mouth
B. Rectum
C. Armpit
D. Groin

74. Rigor mortis in a foetus develops after attaining:
A. 3 months of age
B. 4 months of age
C. 7 months of age
D. 10 months of age

67 A,D 68 A 69 A 70 A 71 A 72 A
73 B 74 C

75. Corpus delicti means:
- **A.** Essence of crime
- **B.** Non decomposed body
- **C.** Identification of dead person
- **D.** Decomposed body

76. Postmortem caloricity is increased in all *except:*
- **A.** Burns
- **B.** Sunstroke
- **C.** Tetanus
- **D.** Septicaemia

77. Algor mortis is:
- **A.** Cadaveric spasm
- **B.** Hypostasis
- **C.** Cooling of body
- **D.** Ethyl alcohol

75 A **76** A **77** C

3

Injuries and Its Medicolegal Importance

- Mechanical injuries (wound) are injuries produced by physical violence.
- **Classification**
  1. *Mechanical:*
     - Abrasions
     - Contusions
     - Lacerations
     - Incised wounds
     - Stab wounds
     - Firearm wounds
     - Fractures and dislocations.
  2. *Thermal:*
     - Due to cold:
       a. Frost bite.
       b. Trench foot.
       c. Immersion foot.
     - Due to heat:
       a. Burns.
       b. Scalds.
  3. *Chemical:*
     a. Corrosive acid.
     b. Corrosive alkalies.
  4. Injuries due to lightning, electricity.

Abrasions (Gravel Rash) Origin: ***ab***-*from and* ***radere***-*to scrape*

- An abrasion is destruction of the skin, which involves superficial layers of epidermis only.
- It has only length and breadth.
  - **Most informative of all injuries.**
- The exposed raw surface is covered by exudation of lymph and blood, which produces a protective covering known as **scab** or **crust (2-3 days).**
- An abrasion may show **"Rolled Edge"** of skin along one side which helps in determining the direction of force.

Types

1. **Scratches:** These are caused by a sharp object passing across the skin, such as fingernails, pin or thorn.
2. **Grazes:** They are most common type* of abrasions. An abrasion caused by violent lateral rubbing by **friction force*** is called **brush burn.** (CF. **Rope burn** is caused by friction of rope against skin leading to blister formation.)
3. **Impact Abrasion:** They are caused by impact of a rough object such as a person is knocked down by a motor car.
4. **Pressure Abrasion:** They are caused by crushing of the superficial layers of the epidermis, e.g., ligature mark of hanging.
   Impact abrasion and pressure abrasions are also known as **Patterned abrasions*.**

Imprint or patterned abrasions may result from forceful impact, as in a pedestrian struck by a vehicle. The importance of patterned abrasions lies in the fact that their shape can be matched to the causative object, and for this reason they should be documented by photography with a scale, or by an accurate tracing. Common examples of imprint abrasions are the sole patterns of footwear in kicking assaults, and motor vehicle or **autorickshaw tyre marks** in run-over pedestrian deaths.

Patterned bruise takes place **rarely** in exceptional cases, when there is immediate death after the injury.

Age of Abrasions*

1. **Fresh**–Bright red.
2. **12 to 24 hours**–Lymph and blood dries up leaving a bright scab.
3. **2 to 3 days–Reddish-brown scab.***
4. **4 to 7 days**–Epithelium grows and covers defect under the scab.
5. **After 7 days**–Scab dries, shrinks and falls out.
   - In **antemortem abrasions,** intravital reaction and congestion is seen.
   - **Erosion** of the skin produced by **ants, excoriations** of the skin by excreta and **pressure sores** can be confused with abrasions.

Contusions (Bruises)

- Origin from the root word **brysan** meaning **to crush.**
  - A contusion is an effusion of blood into the tissues, due to the rupture of the subcutaneous vessels, caused due to violence. Histological Examination shows: **Extravascular RBCs.**
- If the part is vascular and loose, such as **face, vulva, scrotum, a slight degree of violence may cause a large bruise.**
- If the tissues are strongly supported and covered by thick dermis, such as **abdomen,** back, scalp, palm and soles, moderate violence may produce a **small bruise.**
  - Petechiae–pin head size bruise < 2 mm.
- Bruising is more marked on tissues overlying bone in diseased vessels as in arteriosclerosis.
- Children and old people bruise more easily.
- **Stomping**–Kicking and jumping is known as stomping.
- **The Age of Bruise–**A bruise heals by destruction and removal of the extravasated blood.
  1. **At first** (1-2 hours)—Red.
  2. **Few hours to 3 days**—Blue.

3. **4th day—Bluish-black to brown** (hemosiderin).
4. **5 to 6 days**—Greenish (hematoidin).
5. **7 to 12 days**—Yellow (bilirubin).
6. **2 weeks—Normal/Original colour.**

How to remember the sequence of colour change "R VIBGYO*" from "VIBGYO R".

Red
Voilet
Indigo
Brown
Green
Yellow
Original

- Colour change begins from periphery towards centre of bruise [P→C].
- **Subconjunctival Ecchymosis* and Meningeal hemorrhages** do not show colour change.

• In **antemortem bruising,** there is swelling, damage to epithelium, extravasation, coagulation and infiltration of the tissue with blood and colour changes, the margins are NOT sharp*.
  - **Railway Track bruising*:** Caused by whip, or a stick. Mechanism is tractional tear of marginal blood vessels and the central area compresses with no damage.

• Bruises are of **less value** than abrasions because:
1. **Size** of bruise may not correspond to the size of weapon.
2. **Ectopic Bruising**—Site of injury and site of bruise may be different.
   - **Battle's sign*BS:** Bruise of mastoid process due to fracture base of skull in middle cranial fossa. First noted by **Sir Prescott Hewett**. Battle's Sign (BS) tends to be on the side of # (though possible in # on opposite side). Predictive value is 100%.
   - **Racoon sign*RS:** Bilateral periocular bruising due to fracture base of skull in anterior cranial fossa.

Racoon Sign is of less diagnostic value compared with **BS** as **RS** could occur without Skull # (**d/d of RS Amyloid Eye**).

3. Delayed bruising.
4. Bruise do not indicate **direction** of force.

Artificial Bruises: Some irritant substances when applied to skin produce injuries, which simulates bruises, e.g., ***Semicarpus Anacardium (Marking Nut)****, Calotropis.

Incision Test

This test is used to differentiate **bruise from hypostasis.**

- On incision, blood is seen in blood vessel which is **easily washed away in hypostasis.**
- In bruise there is extravasations of blood in surrounding tissue and cannot be washed away.

Incised Wounds

- An **incised wound** is clean cut through the tissues, which is longer than it is deep.
- **Margins are EVERTED.**
- Incised wound appears **lacerated** at scrotum, axilla.
- Incised wounds are **deeper** at their beginning.
- Towards the end of the cut, the wound becomes shallow, called **tailing of the wound,** which indicates direction **(cf.→ FISH TAILING seen in Stab).**
- **Gaping** of incised wound:
  - More when **Langer's lines** have been cut transversely or obliquely.
  - Less when cut Longitudinally (Memorizer **→Langer's-Longitudinal-Less**).
- Incised wounds on ears, nose, genitalia are invariably homicidal in nature. Cuts on genitalia may be result of sexual jealousy, caused by angry paramour, husband or wife.

Age of Incised Wound

1. **Fresh**–Hematoma formation.
2. **12 hours**–Edges are red, swollen and adherent with blood and lymph.
3. **24 hours**–A continuous layer of endothelial cells cover the surface and edges are formed.
4. **36 hours**–The capillary network is complete.
5. **48 to 72 hours**–The wound is filled with fibroblasts.
6. **3 to 5 days**–Definite fibris running parallel to the vessels are seen; vessels show thickening and obliteration.
7. **1 to 2 weeks**–Scar tissue is formed.

   Hesitation marks or **tentative cuts** or **trial wounds**–They are cuts which are multiple, small and superficial, often involving the skin and seen at the beginning of the incised wound. They are seen in **suicidal** wounds.

N.B.→In right-handed persons, self-inflicted injuries are:

- **High on the left side of the neck** and pass downward across the front to end on the right side.
- **Deeper at their origin** and then tail off on the right.

Chop Wound by Axe (SLASH Wound)

Heal end strikes first causing deeper wound, the toe end cause superficial wound, thus helping determine direction of wound and position of assailant.

Stab or Puncture Wounds

- Most important dimension in stab wound is **depth.**
  - DEPTH of Stab Wound:
    - ♦ Less than length of instrument if not fully inserted.
    - ♦ More than length of instrument if fully inserted and body surface compressed, e.g., abdomen, chest.

  - A small penknife can perforate heart or abdominal aorta.
- Punctured wound is deeper than its width and length on skin.
- ***Fish Tailing**** If a *single edged weapon* is used, the surface, triangular, tear drop or wedge shaped, one angle of the wound will be sharp, the other blunt or torn.
- Double edged weapon produce ***Spindle Shaped**** wound.

Potential Question Zone

- A stab wound through the left ventricle of the heart may almost completely seal itself by contraction of the cardiac muscle around the defect. Survival of such a wound is common. A stab wound through the thin-walled **right ventricle**, atrium or coronary is **MORE Fatal.**
- Liver is the most common organ injured in **Direct Stab Injury**
  (Liver > Bowel > Diaphragm > Colon)
- **Violation of Platysma – Penetrating Neck Trauma.**
- **Harakiri *(seppuku):***
  - Traditionally practiced in Japan.
  - Unusual type of suicide.
  - Victim inflicts a stab wound on his abdomen, pulls out intestine.
  - Cause of death is sudden cardiac collapse due to fall in intra-abdominal pressure as a result of sudden evisceration of internal organs (**Syncope**).

Lacerations (From Latin lacerare- to tear)

- Lacerations are tears of skin, mucous membrane muscle or internal organ produced by application of blunt force to the broad area of the body. **Hemorrhage is less profuse compared with incised or stab wounds.**

- **Type of Lacerations**
  1. Split laceration
     – *Incised Like or Incised Looking Wounds:* The sites are the scalp, eyebrows, **cheekbones,** lower jaw, iliac crest, perineum and skin.
  2. Stretch laceration.
  3. **Avulsion laceration** is cause by grinding compression or shearing force at an acute angle to detach a portion of traumatised surface or viscus from its attachments **(Flaying is seen in avulsion laceration. Degloving).**
  4. Tear.
  5. Cut laceration.

Difference Between Incised Looking (Lacerated) and Incised Wound (Magnifying Glass* is Used)

1. In lacerated wound, there are characteristic **Tissue Bridges*** present, when the margins are separated due to crushing of hair bulbs, blood vessels etc.
2. The margins are **irregular with abrasions** as compared to incised wound.

Direction of Force: Lacerations usually curved and the convexity points towards the direction.

Shape of wound may indicate cross-section of instrument.

- Hayfork : Elliptical
- Ice pick : Round
- Poker : Stellate laceration
- File : Triangular laceration
- Scissors : 'Z' shaped

Defence Wounds (DW)

- It results due to immediate and instinctive reaction of the victim to save himself, either by raising the arm to prevent the attack or by grasping the weapon.

Common Sites of DW:
- Extensor surface of the forearms (the ulnar side).
- Lateral/posterior aspects of the upper arm.
- Dorsum of the hands.
- Outer and posterior aspects of lower limbs and back.

Fabricated wounds (fictitious, forged or invented wound).

Self-inflicted wounds:
- Are those inflicted by a person on his own body.

Self-suffered wound:
- Are those, which may be produced by another person with one's consent.

Regional Injuries

Fracture Skull

- Most fragile bone in the skull to get fractured is– temporal.
  1. **Linear or fissured fractures:**
     - Most common type of skull fracture or cracks in the bone, involving entire thickness of bone, or outer or inner table only.
  2. Depressed fracture is also called **Signature fracture.**
     - Localized depressed fracture is caused by blows from heavy weapon with a small striking surface, e.g., stone, stick, axe, hammer, etc.
     - The outer table is driven into the diploe, inner table is fractured irregularly.

     Depressed skull # is NOT always over the immediate area of impact of brain.
  3. **Pond or indented fractures:** They occur only in skulls, which are elastic, i.e., the skulls of **infants.**
  4. **Gutter fractures:** They are formed when part of the thickness of the bone is removed so as to form a gutter, e.g., oblique bullet wound.
  5. **Comminuted fracture:** Multiple fracture of skull, also called **Spider web fracture.**

COUP VS CONTRECOUP INJURIES
(Focal Brain Injuries)

Coup Injury: Occurs under the site of impact with an object, when a moving object impacts the stationary head.
Mechanism: The skull is temporarily bent inward and impacts the brain. Direct Injury.
Contrecoup Injury: Occurs on the side opposite the area that was hit, when the moving head strikes a stationary object. Indirect Injury. First described by **Jean Louis Petit.**
Mechanism: Contrecoup lesions are result of **abrupt deceleration of the head**, causing the brain to collide with the inside of the skull. CSF is denser than the brain, rushes to the area of impact during the injury, forcing the brain back into the other side of the skull. *Examples:* Shaken Baby syndrome and Vehicle Accidents. **Traumatic Lens Dislocation** unusual example.
PQZ→ Contrecoup is least **likely to occur in forward fall** because in forward fall brain hits the posterior cranial floor and wall which have smoother interiors! And more common over the **frontal and temporal poles** where skull surface is rough.

Cerebral Contusion

(Most common sites Frontal lobe and Temporal lobe)

- **Intermediary Coup:** Contusion of the deep brain structures.
- **Gliding Contusions:** Contusion of the Dorsal surface of the cerebral hemispheres.
- **Plaque Jaune:** Old Cortical Contusion may resolve/heal as a **yellow** lesion (also known as *plaque jaune*) in the brain, normally seen at the inferior aspect of the frontal lobe.
- **Concussion** is a state of temporary unconsciousness, which results from violence applied to the skull. ***Berlin's oedema*** is seen in concussion.

– Concussions of the spinal cord is called **railway spine.**

Retraction Balls*: The forces generated by violent shaking or rotational injury (as in a passenger ejected from a moving vehicle) can produce stretching of axons in cerebral white matter. The force may be strong enough to shear off axons, the ends of which retract into globoid shapes that appear with **silver stain of white matter as "retraction balls"**.

After 12 hours anatomical injuries to axon begins to become visible.

Sequence

Sausage links (dilated)→Club Shaped→Round balls known as Retraction Balls. Retraction balls represent **"transected" axon** (could be brain or spinal cord or both*).

(N.B. → Spontaneous Splenic Rupture may occur with Mononucleosis, Leukemia or Malaria).

Pedestrians injuries are classified into:

Primary Impact Injuries:

- Produced on the part of the body which is first contacted by the vehicle.
- ***Bumper fracture is wedge shaped*** fracture of the tibia and fibula, if a person is hit from behind when both feet are well fixed on the ground.
- These are often patterned injuries.

Secondary Impact Injuries:

Produced by a subsequent contact of the victim with the vehicle as it happens when he is thrown **on to the vehicle** or when the vehicle runs over the victim.

Secondary injuries (also called Tertiary* impact injuries): Are produced due to the effects of fall when coming in **contact with the ground**.

These injuries are usually seen over the prominent parts of the body viz. knee, hips.

Three scenarios depending on where the vehicle hits wrt. Center of Gravity (CoG)

1. Impact **below** CoG throws victim on to bonnet (or roof at greater speed).
2. Impact **at** CoG: Victim thrown in direction of travel.
3. Impact **above** CoG: Throws victim under vehicle.
   - **Seatbelt Injury:** Most common injury due to seatbelt is rupture of small bowel and associated injury to **mesentery.**
   - **Motorcyclist's Fracture:** Base of skull, the middle cranial fossa fractures traversed the sphenoid in the region of spheno-occipital synchondrosis. **Hinge Fracture*.**
   - **Sparrow's foot marks** are bizarre shaped lacerations that result when the face coming in contact with **shattered windshield glass**. It is a commonly seen in front seat passengers in road traffic.

     [***Be-aware: Don't Confuse CROW FEET SIGN with Sparrow's Feet (Windshield Injury)***

     Radial bands beside the eyes—so called "crow's feet" which are *absence of burns and soot deposits at the corner of eye*. The heat and metallic deposits may also lead to a *crow's feet*-like pattern around the eyes.

     They are a sign of **vital reaction** in the cases of traumatic and thermic injury, possibly also in high-voltage burns due to sparking.

     Clue to "Flash Fires", Explosive Injuries: The injury is due to convicted rather than radiant energy.

     In general, the "crow's feet" show that the person was conscious at the moment of the event.]

- **Whiplash injury** is due to the violent acceleration or deceleration force. There is hyperflexion followed by acute hyperextension. **Hyper-extension (main injury)** causes injury to cervical column especially lower cervical region.

- In **Boxing injuries**–fracture of the skull is rare but **subdural hemorrhage** occurs most common type of hemorrhage, it can lead to parkinson's disease like symptom called or *Dementia pugilistica** or *Punch-Drunk syndrome.*
  - **Deterioration of speed and co-ordination** are the chief symptoms of the onset of punch-drunk (traumatic encephalopathy) condition.
  - Repeated blows to the head produce small hemorrhages and degenerative changes in brain.

Fracture of Bone

- Antemortem fractures have blood effusion, laceration edema which is not seen in postmortem fracture.
  - Provisional callus formation tubes 1 week.
  - Callus formation takes 3 weeks.

Callus is converted into hard bones in 2 months.

Intracranial Hemorrhage

1. **Extradural Hemorrhage**
   - It is caused always due to trauma. (Least common type of I/C Hemorrhage).
   - Most common artery causing extradural hemorrhage is **anterior branch of middle meningeal artery.**
   - There is a history of head injury, which causes the bleeding and will usually cause temporary unconsciousness. This is followed by a period of normal consciousness, the **lucid interval*** of few hours to a week.
   - Radiology: Biconvex appearance.
   - Heat haematoma resembles extradural hemorrhage.

2. Subdural Hemorrhage

- Most common intracranial hemorrhage due to head injury.
- May occur from relatively small amount of trauma.
  - It occurs due to rupture of bridging veins.
- Subdural hemorrhage is seen in:
  - Punch-drunk syndrome
  - Chronic alcoholics
  - Old age
  - Infantile whiplash syndrome.
- Death may occur if hemorrhage exceeds 50 ml.
- **Pachy Meningitis Hemorrhagica:** It is a chronic subdural hemorrhage.
- Subdural hygroma*
  - Accumulation of CSF in subdural space due to rupture of arachnoid layer.*
- **Radiology:** Crescent Shape.

3. Subarachnoid Hemorrhage

- It is essentially venous or capillary, not arterial.
- Most common site of rupture of Berry Aneurysm is *Anterior Communicated artery. Vertebral Artery least common site.*
- Most common cause of subarachnoid hemorrhage is trauma.*

Subdural v/s Subarachnoid Blood
Subdural blood will not coat the brain surface and follow the contours (as with subarachnoid hemorrhage), but rather will fall off the brain when the skull is opened. Sometimes subdural blood will adhere to the skull cap which can also differentiate it from subarachnoid blood. Subdural blood will **wash away under running water** whereas S/arachnoid blood will remain intact.

4. **Intracerebral Hemorrhage**
   Most common non-traumatic hemorrage
   Most common site of intracerebral hemorrhage is internal capsule, at lenticulostraite branch of middle cerebral artery **(Charcoit's artery). Intra-Parenchymal Hemorrhage, most common type of I/C Hemorrhage (Hyper-tension).**
   Site of Hemorrhage following Head Injury: Intra-Parenchymal, Subarachnoid, Subdural, Epidural spaces.
   Duret Hemorrhages*: Delayed secondary hemorrhages in mid-brain and pons.

Firearm Injuries

Forensic Ballistics (FB) is the science dealing with the investigation of firearms, ammunition the motion of projectiles, i.e., bullets and the problem arising from their use.

Classification

a. **Internal ballistics:** The study of projectiles in the weapon.
b. **External ballistics:** The behaviour of the projectile through air.
c. **Terminal ballistics:** The study of the penetration of a medium denser than air by projectiles.
   1. Sub category of terminal ballistics, is **Wound Ballistics**, is primarily concerned with the penetration, motion and effects of missiles on body (**Domain of Forensic Pathologist***).

"Some High School Physics": The amount of tissue damage is determined by the amount of kinetic energy lost by the projectile in the body. Kinetic energy is illustrated as **KE = W×V×V/2g**, where: W=bullet weight, V=velocity, g=gravitational acceleration. **Bullet velocity** being the **most critical component.**

There are three mechanisms of tissue damage due to bullets:

i. **Laceration and Crushing:** Generated by the projectile displacing the tissues in its track and are recognized as the primary wounding mechanism produced by handguns.

ii. **Shock Waves:** Compression of tissues that lay ahead of the bullet, are generated by high velocity missiles.

iii. **Cavitation:** When a missile enters the body, the kinetic energy imparted on the surrounding tissues forces them forward and radially producing a temporary cavity or temporary displacement of tissues.

General Considerations

1. Wounding capacity of a **missile striking bone will be greater than in soft tissues**, as bone acts as a superior retardant force that is more effective at decelerating a projectile and increasing the energy transfer than less compact substances.
2. **Cancellous bone,** the spongy bone found on the epiphyses of long bones, will experience **less damage** than the **more compact cortical bone**, because the KE can more readily dissipate within the honeycomb structures of the cancellous bone. **Bu(T)Terfly** fracture is seen in **(T)Tibia** due to firearm injury.
3. **Bevelling of the skull in bullet injury:** The principle which guides the occurrence of bevelling is that the bullet produce bevelling in the second layer (or exit point).
   - *In entry wound* the bevelling is present in inner table of skull.
   - *In exit wound* the bevelling is present in the outer table of skull. **Absence of abrasion** at wound margin is **diagnostic of exit wound.**

The **entrance wound** is circular, with inverted edges and is surrounded by blackened and singed area.

Bevelling vs. Punched Out

When a bullet enters the skull it produces a sharp-edged **"punched out" hole in the outer table**, with a larger corresponding "beveled-out" hole on the inner table. As the bullet exits the cranial cavity, the inner table appears "punched out" with bevelling on the outer table.

Back-Spatter: Clothes, hair, tissue may enter the muzzle end, due to negative pressure.

Shored Exit Wound is An Atypical Exit Wounds with surrounding area of **Abrasion**. When the bullet exits through skin pressed against a firm object, such as a belt or backrest of a chair.

Comparison of Rifled Weapon with Smooth Bored Weapon (Shotgun)

1. In rifled firearm there are groove and lands present in the bore.

   In shot gun the bore is smooth*.
2. The projectile in the cartridge of rifled weapon is bullet*.

   The projectile in the cartridge of shot gun are short pellets.*

   Cartridge of shot gun has:
   1. Felt wad (helps lubrication, sealing of bore, separate propellant from projectiles).
   2. Detonator cap (zinc or copper).
   3. Cardboard or plastic disc.

Advantages of Rifling

- Gives spin and rotation to bullet.
- Increase accuracy and range.
- Checks wobbling.
- Enhance wounding power.
- Provides Gyroscopic stability.

Some Important Concepts in Forensic Ballistics

a. **Calibre**

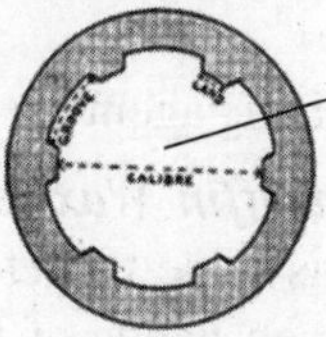	Calibre is the distance between two diagonally **opposite lands** used for only rifled firearms*

b. **Bore of gun/Gauge of gun**
- Used only in context of shot gun.
- Number of balls/pellets of equal size and weight as can be made from 454 gms (1 pound) of lead*.
- Bore determines the size of pellets*.

c. **Choking** is a constricting device at the **muzzle end** of the **shot gun.*** The purpose of choking is to lessen the rate of spread of shot after it leaves the muzzle. (c.f. choking in mechanical asphyxia).
Paradox Gun*—When the muzzle end of the shot gun is rifled it is called Paradox gun.

d. **Revolver**
- It has a cylindrical magazine situated at the back of the barrel, which is capable of revolving motion. The empty cartridge remains inside revolver (Revolver never ejects cartridges automatically*).
- The range of revolver is 100 m.

e. **Air rifle and Air pistol**
- In these, compressed air is used to fire lead sluds.
- Empty cartridges an ejected out from automatic pistol.

f. **Primer**
- Lead Styphnate, Tetrazene, Barium Nitrate, Antimony Sulphide are used as primers.
- They on pressure detonates and ignite gun powder.

g. **Powders**

- **Black gun powder**–It consists of **potassium nitrate 75%, sulphur 10%, and charcoal 15%.**

  Use of Constituent:

  – Potassium nitrate—Oxidising agent

  [*Dermal Nitrate Test/Paraffin Wax test/ Diphenyl Amine Test** is done to detect presence of gun powder on hands of the person who has fired the gun].

  – Sulphur—Increase density by acting as binding agent.

  – Charcoal—Fuel.

  [**N.B.: FG "Fine Grain"** denotes the **fineness** of Gun Powder particles, moreFs quicker it will burn.]

- **Smokeless**

  *Nitrocellulose (single base).

  **Nitroglycerine and nitrocellulose (double base).

  ***With nitro guanidine*(triple base) powder.

  It produces much less flame and smoke and are more completely burnt than black powder.

Ballistic Coefficient (c) → c = m/i × d^2

The ballistics coefficient of a projectile depicts its capacity to maintain its velocity against air resistance. It is a relationship between mass (m), diameter (d), and a form factor (i) determined by the shape of the bullet.

C = mass/form factor × (diameter)^2

N.B. → A larger ballistics coefficient means projectile move more effectively and lose less velocity as they travel.

Firearm Discharge Residue

- Primer → Lead, Antimony, Barium
- Powder → Nitrocellulose, Nitroglycerine, Nitroguanidine
- Bullet → Lead, copper, iron
- Cartridge → Copper, zinc, nickel
- Barrel → Iron, Petroleum products

Infrared spectra can provide a total chemical picture of the weapon. Gun powder from different manufacturers and suppliers, for example, may have different chemical formulations. Gun powder on blood stained clothing thus can be visualized by IR Rays.

Infrared Photography: Forensic Applications

- Document examinations:
  - Reveal writing, printing, or other markings under obliteration on documents.
  - Illegible charred, aged or worn documents can often be rendered legible in infrared photographs.
  - Erased writing.
- Dyes used in cloth and the physical properties of the cloth.
- Presence of stains *is an excellent application for infrared reflected photography.*
- Blood stain pattern examination.
- Gun shot residue detection.
- Bite marks examination.

Detection of Gun Shot Residues:

- Dermal Nitrate Test.
- Harrison and Gilroy Test.
- Neutron Activation Analysis.
- Atomic Absorption Spectroscopy.
- Flameless Atomic Absorption Spectroscopy.
- Scanning electron microscope-energy dispersive X-ray analysis (SED-EDXA).

h. **Bullets**

- Bullet is made up of lead.
- The extent of muscle damage by a bullet depends primarily on the **velocity.**
- Large round bullet causes greater damage to the body.
- A bullet is picked up with hands.
- **A DumDum Bullet also known as Expanding Bullet,** so called because tip is chiseled out, is one, which fragments extensively upon striking, cause extensive damage (name comes from a place near Kolkata).
- **Express bullet**—Bullet in which a hole is present.
- **Tracer bullet**—Powder in the base so that it burns brightly*.
- **Incendiary bullets** contain phosphorus.
- **Souvenir bullet**—When the bullet remains in body for a long period of time is called souvenir bullet. It causes chronic lead poisoning.
- **Glance bullet** causes gutter fracture.
- **Mushrooming of Bullet:** A bullet with a soft nose, after hitting the target gets deformed into mushroom like shape.
- **Piggyback bullet** —When bullet fails to come out from muzzy, this bullet is pushed by another bullet (piggy back bullet). In *Tandem cartridge* 2 bullets are present in same cartridge which enters the target at different points.

i. **Wounds from shot-gun (Suggesting Range)**

Shape of wound	*Distance*
1. Cruciate or Stellate shape	Contact over bone
2. Oval shape	Upto 30 cm
3. Rat hole wound	30-100 cm
4. Satellite wound	More than 2 metres
5. Individual pellets	Over 4 metres

j. **Products of Firing from Rifled Firearms (Suggesting Range)**

Tattooing (Antemortem Stippling/Peppering)

- Deposition of unburnt powder particles **cannot be wiped** away.
- Tattooing is the sine qua non of **Intermediate*** Range Firearm Injury.

Blackening (Smudging)

- Black smoke of burnt powder can be wiped away.
- Blackening is seen at distance closer than tattooing.

Singeing and Scorching

- It is produced by heat and flames.
- Scorching and singeing are seen at distance closer than blackening.

  [**Memorizer:** Remember the word "**T**u**B**erculo**S**i**S**" to remember relative distance from wound].

k. **Kennedy's Phenomenon**—Due to surgical alteration evaluation of wound as entry or exit wound becomes difficult.

l. A bullet is picked up with **hands** because fired bullet has Primary Markings (**Class Characteristics**) and Secondary Markings (**Individual Characteristics***) which may be altered using metallic instruments.

m. **Markings in Bullet**

1. **Primary markings:**
   - It is called **class** characteristic.
   - It results from manufacturing specifications, design and dimensions of gun, helps in identification of gun.
2. **Secondary markings:**
   - It is called **individual** characteristics.
   - It tells about individual gun, the irregularities are caused by sticking of the particles of bullet to bore when shots are fired also known as ***Metal Fouling****.

Atypical entrance wounds are caused because of:

- **Yaw:** Deviation between long axis of bullet and the axis of path.
- **Tumbling:** Rotation of bullet end to end.
- **Wobbling:** Few micro-seconds after bullet leaves muzzle.
- **Slap:** When bullet strikes the skin at very acute angle, and doesn't perforate the skin.
- **Richochet:** Rebound, deviation, deflection of bullet after striking intermediate object.
  [**Keyhole Defect:** A missile striking the skull tangentially, as may occur in graze wounds, produces a keyhole defect (**Ricochet and Yawning Bullet**) In the keyhole lesion, one end of the perforation will resemble a typical entrance defect, while the other end will show external bevelling consistent exit holes also known as **Gutter Wound**.]

Abraded collar and grease or dirt collar are present in gun shot **entrance** injury, tells about the direction*.

- **Puppe's Rule:** Puppe's rule help assess the chronological order in which fractures were formed, since later fractures will typically stop at previously formed ones. The short fracture lines from the exit wound stop at the previously formed entrance wound fractures. Helps in determining the sequence of bullets to hit the skull, when there are multiple bullet injuries in skull.
- **Cancellous bone, the spongy bone** found on the epiphyses of long bones, will experience **less damage** than the **more compact cortical bone**, because the KE can more readily dissipate within the honeycomb structures of the cancellous bone.

n. **Rayalasima Phenomenon:**

A person killed by stab injury and then bullet is implanted inside to, mislead investigation.

o. **Bullet Auditing (Matching bullets with wounds)**

Baseline Rule: Number of entrance wounds = Number of exit wounds.

Exceptions:

a. Bullets are still in the body.
b. Tandem bullets – 2 bullets entered (or exited) at the same place.
c. Secondary projectile – a bullet hit a bone, and made it fly out of the body.

Hidden Entrance/Exit wounds: Below Chin, Inside mouth, Ears, Back, Anus.

BLAST INJURIES

Other terms used, particularly for **Air Blast**, are:

- Blast concussion and reflex paralysis, blast chest, shell shock.
- Vent du boulet, Wind of shot, Breath of the cannon ball.

There are 4 types of blast injury and an individual patient may be injured by more than one mechanism:

- **Primary:** Injury from over-pressurization force (**blast/shock waves**) impacting the body surface.
  - TM rupture, pulmonary damage and air embolization, hollow viscus injury.
- **Secondary:** Injury from projectiles (bomb fragments, flying debris).
  - Penetrating trauma, fragmentation injuries, blunt trauma.
- **Tertiary:** Injuries from displacement of victim by the **blast wind.**
  - Blunt/penetrating trauma, fractures and traumatic amputations.
- **Quaternary:** All other injuries from the blast.
  - Crush injuries, burns, asphyxia, toxic exposures, exacerbations of chronic illness.

Primary Blast Injuries: The pressure wave hits the body, and while most of it is reflected, some of it manages to compress internal gases. As a result, the victim sustains **primary blast injuries**.

Main mechanisms involved in the pathogenesis of primary blast injuries:

1. Spalling (Turbulence at Air/liquid interface) **[POTENTIAL Q. Zone].**
2. Implosion.
3. Inertia.
4. And pressure differentials.

These typically affect ***ears* (Tympanic membrane most common primary blast injury)*, the lungs, and — in rare cases — intestines*** (esp. colon*). These gassy chambers basically implode, rupturing and fragmenting tissue.

Blast lungs refers to severe pulmonary contusion, bleeding or swelling with damage to alveoli and blood vessels, or a combination of these. Characterized by areas of blotchy purple-black sub-pleural hemorrhage. It is the **most common cause of death** among people who initially survive an explosion.

CXR: "Butterfly" pattern.**

In air the gas and air surrounding the explosion are compressed and absorb energy from the explosion.

In water, being incompressible, there is little absorption and the pressure wave is transmitted with greater intensity over a longer range.

The **lethal range of an explosion in water is far greater than the same mass of explosion in air** and this increases mortality in underwater explosions.

Most Severely Affected Organs:**

Air Blast: Lungs.

Underwater: G.I.T.

Most Common:

Air: Tympanic membrane.

Underwater (fully submerged) T.M.

Underwater (Head is out) G.I.T.

Molotov cocktail is also known as a petrol bomb or alcohol bomb (NB→Not a poison*).

It is a simple type of **improvised incendiary device**, consists of a stoppered bottle filled with a combustible liquid, such as gasoline or high-proof alcohol, with a fuel-soaked rag stuffed in the neck of the bottle.

Marshall's triad: Punctate bruises, abrasions and lacerations, seen in explosion injuries.

MEDICOLEGAL IMPORTANCE OF INJURIES

Important Definitions

1. **Injury:** Any harm whatever illegally caused in Body, Mind, Reputation or Property (Memory Aid → **BMR** is an important concept of **P**hysiology).
   - Section Forty-four (44), IPC.
2. **Murder:** Definition is under section 300 IPC and punishment under Section 302 IPC.

Doctrine of Diminished Responsibility and Section 300 of IPC

In India, Doctrine of Diminished Responsibility is used only in murder cases to reduce the charge to manslaughter, i.e., Exceptions 1 and 4 of Section 300 of IPC.

Exception 1.—When culpable homicide is not murder.—Culpable homicide is not murder if the offender, whilst deprived of the power of self-control by grave and sudden provocation, causes the death of the person who gave the provocation or causes the death of any other person by mistake or accident.

The above exception is subject to the following provisos:

- First—That the provocation is not sought or voluntarily provoked by the offender as an excuse for killing or doing harm to any person.
- Secondly—That the provocation is not given by anything done in obedience to the law, or

by a public servant in the lawful exercise of the powers of such public servant.

- Thirdly—That the provocation is not given by anything done in the lawful exercise of the right of private defence.

Exception 4.—Culpable homicide is not murder if it is committed without premeditation in a sudden fight in the heat of passion upon a sudden quarrel and without the offender having taken undue advantage or acted in a cruel or unusual manner.

Explanation—It is immaterial in such cases which party offers the provocation or commits the first assault.

3. **Hurt:**
   - Section 319 (IPC).
   - **B**odily pain, **D**isease or **In**firmity caused to a person **(BID).**
4. **Grievous Hurt:**
   - According to **S 320 I.P.C. (Only Defines*)** any of the following injury is grievous: The eight clauses of grievous injury can be remembered with the help of sentence **Memorizer→** "**E**very **S**tudent **H**as re**MEMBER**ed **I**njury's **D**efinition and **F**orgot it within **20 days** of **P**assing **E**xams".
     1. **Emasculation** (Impotency/sterility).
     2. Permanent privation (loss) of **Sight** of either eye.
     3. Permanent privation of **Hearing** of either ear.
     4. Privatation of any **Member or joint.**
     5. Destruction or permanent **Impairing** of the power of any member or joint.
     6. Permanent **Disfiguration** of the head and face.
     7. **Fracture** or dislocation **of a bone or tooth (Discontinuity till medullary cavity is considered grievous).**

8. Any hurt which **Endangers** life or, which causes the victim to be in the **severe bodily Pain** or unable to follow his *ordinary pursuits* (not mere hospitalization) for **a period of 20 days.**

5. **Dangerous Weapon*(Sec 324 and Sec 326 IPC):** Any weapon used for Stabbing Shooting or Cutting **(S.S.C.), or is likely to cause death.**
6. **Sequence of enzymes/biochemical markers rising after injury:**
   - Tissue cathepsin (5-10 min).
   - Seretonin (10 min).
   - Histamines (20-30 min).
   - Esterase and ATPase (within 1 hour).
   - Aminopeptidase (2 hours).
   - Acid phosphatase (4 hours).
   - Alkaline phosphatase (6 hours).
7. **Ewing's Postulates (AIIMS 2015)**
   These postulates should be satisfied before a relationship between ***Trauma and New growth*** is accepted.
   1. Evidence of previous **integrity** of the injured part.
   2. **Undeniable and Adequate** trauma must be proved.
   3. There must be a proof of reasonable **time interval** between injury and appearance of tumor.
   4. Disease must develop at the **exact site** of injury.
   5. The **nature** of the tumour must be proved.
8. **Raekillo** conducted the study to find out histochemical changes in wounds.
9. **Rose System** used for depicting injuries on Medicolegal report.
   - **Incised Wounds:** One red line.
   - **Abrasions:** Multiple closely spaced red lines (**Red hatching**).
   - **Contusions:** Multiple closely-spaced blue lines (**Blue hatching**).

   [Neel (Blue) – Contusion]

MCQs

1. **Minimal air resulting in fatal pulmonary embolism is:**
   A. 25 ml B. 50 ml
   C. 100 ml D. 200 ml
2. **Following are grievous injuries *except:***
   A. Emasculation
   B. Dislocation of tooth
   C. Chopping of a finger
   D. Admission for 20 days in a hospital
3. **Section of IPC dealing with grievous hurt is:**
   A. 319 IPC B. 320 IPC
   C. 323 IPC D. 325 IPC
4. **Amount of blood present in an adult in relation to his body weight is:**
   A. 2-3% B. 5-6%
   C. 10-12% D. 15%
5. **Enzyme showing increase after an hour of sustaining injury is:**
   A. Aminopeptidase
   B. Acid phosphatase
   C. Alkaline phosphatase
   D. Esterase
6. **Provisional callus (in a fractured bone) starts forming from:**
   A. 1st day onwards B. 3rd day onwards
   C. 14th day onwards D. 6th week onwards
7. **Suicidal nature of cut throat injuries are indicated by:**
   A. Horizontally placed cut
   B. Multiple irregularly placed cuts
   C. Tentative cuts
   D. Cuts present below thyroid cartilage

1 C 2 D 3 B 4 B 5 D 6 B 7 C

8. Knocked out tooth socket is filled up with soft tissues by:

A. 1 day **B.** 1 week
C. 2 weeks **D.** 1 month

9. Cause of death in crush syndrome is:

A. Fat embolism
B. Muscle necrosis
C. Infection/septicamia
D. Acute renal failure

10. Edges of incised wound are normally formed by:

A. 12 hours **B.** 24 hours
C. 3 days **D.** 7 days

11. Grievous injury includes which of the following?

A. Incised wound of scalp
B. Lacerated wound of scalp
C. Fracture radius
D. Injury which kept patient away from work for 10 days
E. Abdominal trauma

12. Bevelling of the skull is seen in:

A. Broad end of the entry point in bullet injury
B. Narrow end of the entry point in bullet injury
C. Exit point of bullet
D. Depressed fracture of the skull

13. Grease colour is seen with .... wounds.

A. Firearm entry
B. Firearm exit
C. Road traffic accident
D. Hanging

14. Joule burn is seen with:

A. Electrocution
B. Scalds
C. Lighting
D. Vitroilage

---

8 B 9 D 10 B 11 C 12 C 13 A 14 A

15. Which of the following constitute grievous injury?
A. Incised wound of scalp
B. Incised wound of thigh
C. Fracture tibia
D. Laceration of the scalp

16. Grease colour is seen with:
A. Electrocution
B. Lightning
C. Thermal injury
D. Bullet entry

17. In a lacerated wound the hair bulb is:
A. Cut
B. Crushed
C. Both of the above
D. Lacerated

18. Where does a lacerated wound appear like an incised wound?
A. Abdomen
B. Thorax
C. Hand
D. Forehead

19. Gutter fracture result from:
A. Injury with a large round object
B. Bullet injuries
C. Automobile accident
D. Falling from a height

20. Grievous injury includes all *except*:
A. Emasculisation
B. Loss of 15 days work
C. Permanent disfigurement
D. Fracture of bones
E. All of the above

21. Privation of any member of joint is a .....hurt.
A. Simple
B. Grievous
C. Serious
D. Dangerous

22. Greenish colour in a contusion is due to:
A. Hemosiderin
B. Haematoidin
C. Bilirubin
D. Biliverdin

---

15 C 16 D 17 B 18 D 19 B 20 B 21 B 22 B

23. Tentative cuts occur in which injury?

A. Accidental **B.** Suicidal

C. Homicidal **D.** Fabricated

24. Markings in a projectile occurs in:

A. Double barrel gun

B. Pistol

C. Rifle

D. Shot gun

25. Which is true about stab wound?

A. Breath is maximum

B. Length is maximum

C. Depth is maximum

D. It has wound of entry and exit

26. Dermal nitrate test detects:

A. Nitrite salt poisoning

B. Blood stains

C. Nerve gas poisoning

D. Gun powder residue

27. Postmortem wound best differs from the antemortem wound by:

A. Gaps on incising

B. No clots

C. Absence of erythema and cellular changes

D. Stain can be removed by washing

28. Which of the following indicates that the wound in a hospitalized woman typist hit by lathis admitted for 20 days was grievous?

A. She is not able to be recognized

B. Wound does not heal completely

C. Incised wound over scalp

D. She is not able to do her daily routines

29. A clean incised wound heals by:

A. Primary intention

B. Secondary intention

C. Excessive scarring

D. None of the above

23 B 24 C 25 C 26 D 27 C 28 D 29 A

30. Tearing of the skin and subcutaneous tissue is called:

A. Abrasion
B. Laceration
C. Contusion
D. Avulsions

31. On tenth day of a tooth being knocked out, the local clinical finding will be:

A. Tooth socket being filled up by tissue
B. Blood, clots in the socket
C. Alveolar process smooth
D. Fluid blood in the socket

32. The effective range of shot gun is:

A. 10 to 15 yards
B. 20 to 30 yards
C. 30 to 40 yards
D. 60 to 80 yards

33. False vesication differs from true vesication *except:*

A. Produced after death
B. Vesicles contain gas and no fluid
C. No inflammatory or respiratory zone present
D. None of the above

34. Dowry death is included in the following section of the Indian Penal Code:

A. 304-A
B. 304-B
C. 320
D. 498-A

35. Bullet is picked up with:

A. Toothed forceps
B. Hands
C. Scissors
D. Needle

36. Spinal cord is opened from the:

A. Frontal approach
B. Back side
C. Lateral side
D. None of the above

30 B 31 A 32 C 33 D 34 B 35 B 36 B

37. Compressed air is used to fire lead slugs in:

A. Automatic pistol
B. Revolver
C. Air rifle
D. Shot gun

38. Detonator cap is situated at:

A. Top of the bullet
B. Side of the bullet case
C. Base of the rim
D. None of them

39. Section 302 of Indian Penal Code is for:

A. Rape
B. Murder
C. Grievous hurt
D. Attempt to commit suicide

40. Pellet holes in a firearm wound is seen if distance is:

A. 60 cm **B.** 100 cm
C. 150 cm **D.** 200 cm

41. Incised like lacerated wound appears at:

A. Forehead
B. Hand
C. Thorax
D. Abdomen

42. One of the following substances produce injuries which stimulate contusion:

A. Semicarpus anacardium
B. Ricinus communis
C. Abrus precatorius
D. Capsicum annum

43. Smokeless gun powder is composed of:

A. $KMnO_4$
B. HCN
C. Nitrocellulose
D. Sulphur

37 C 38 C 39 B 40 D 41 A 42 A 43 C

44. Mercury fulminate is used in firearm ammunition as:

A. Detonator
B. Smokeless powder
C. Black powder
D. Mixed powder

45. 'Pond Fracture' is seen commonly in:

A. Persons who are over 50 years of age
B. Young adults
C. Children
D. Women

46. Full dispersion is seen in:

A. Full choked
B. Half choked
C. Unchoked
D. All of the above

47. Choking is a constricting device within the barrel at the muzzle end of:

A. Revolver
B. 303 rifle
C. Shot gun
D. Semiautomatic pistol

48. "Fracture a-la signature" is:

A. A depressed fracture
B. A fissured fracture
C. Separation of the suture lines
D. A ring fracture

49. Open wound is a ....

A. Contusion
B. Abrasion
C. Laceration
D. Concussion

50. Brush injury is due to:

A. Friction
B. Electric shock
C. Scalds
D. Bullet injury

---

44 A 45 C 46 C 47 C 48 A 49 C 50 A

51. One of the following is an example of a grievous injury:
A. Scalp laceration
B. Forearm laceration requiring and stitches
C. Fracture of radius
D. Groin injury with loss of 1 litre of blood

52. The most common type of haemorrhage in injury to boxers is:
A. Extradural
B. Subdural
C. Intracerebral
D. Intraventricular

53. Which is not true regarding colour of bruise?
A. 4th day–bruise black to brown
B. 7-12 days–green
C. 1st day–red
D. 2 Weeks–normal

54. All are components of black gun powder *except:*
A. Sulphur
B. Charcoal
C. Potassium nitrate
D. Lead peroxide

55. Postmortem autopsy is done for:
A. Whole body
B. Parts which are injured
C. Parts which have been asked for an inquest
D. Parts which relatives have given permission for

56. In deep incised wounds, Langer's lines determine:
A. Direction
B. Gaping
C. Shelving
D. Healing

57. Damage produced by a bullet fired from a person is in direct proportion of its:
A. Size
B. Shape
C. Velocity
D. Weight

58. Which is associated with shotgun alone?
A. Gun powder
B. Primer
C. Projectile
D. Wads

---

51 C 52 B 53 B 54 D 55 A 56 B 57 D 58 D

59. For dowry death punishment is:
A. 3-year imprisonment + Rs. 10,000/-
B. 5-year imprisonment + Rs. 15,000/-
C. 7-year imprisonment + Rs. 20,000/-
D. 2-year imprisonment + Rs. 15,000/-

60. Grievous hurt is punishable under section ………… IPC.
A. 320 B. 354
C. 321 D. 402

61. Negligence on the part of the father towards the son can be punished under section:
A. 319 B. 317
C. 315 D. 318

62. Which of the following sections of IPC are concerned with dowry death?
A. 300 B. 302
C. 304 D. 304-A
E. 304-B

63. Grievous injury includes all of the following *except:*
A. Emasculation
B. Permanent privation of hearing
C. Privation of any member/joint
D. Disability to follow one's ordinary pursuits for a period of a week
E. Permanent disfiguration of face

64. Dermal nitrate test is done for the detection of:
A. Gun powder residue B. Seminal stains
D. Saliva C. Blood stains

65. Puppe's rule is related to:
A. Sequence of bullets
B. Enzyme assay in blisters
C. Related to age estimation
D. Sex determination

59 C 60 A 61 B 62 E 63 D 64 A 65 A

66. Gutter fracture is due to:
A. A sharp weapon
B. Firearm injury
C. Blunt weapon
D. Serrated edge

67. Detection of metals (heavy) is done by using all tests *except:*
A. Harrison-Gilroy test
B. Spectroscopic examination
C. Neutron activation test
D. Paraffin test

68. Black gun powder; ingredient not present is:
A. Sulphur
B. Arsenic
C. Charcoal
D. Potassium nitrate

69. I.P.C. section for grievous injury:
A. Section 420 B. Section 320
C. Section 299 D. Section 351

70. Blackening and tattooing of skin and clothing can be best demonstrated by:
A. Luminol spray
B. Infra red photography
C. Ultraviolet light
D. Magnifying lens

71. Antemortem of blister differs from postmortem blister by:
A. Presence of albumin and chloride in blister fluid
B. Gas in blister
C. Dry hard surface of the floor of blister (punctured)
D. Absence of hyperemia around the blister

66 B 67 D 68 B 69 B 70 B 71 A

72. Injury means harm caused illegally to a person in:
A. Body B. Property
C. Reputation D. All of the above

73. Incised looking wound is:
A. Avulsion laceration B. Tear laceration
C. Cut laceration D. Split laceration

74. A brush burn is:
A. Electric burn B. Arborasent mark
C. Grazed abrasion D. Impact abrasion

75. Scab is formed over an abrasion in about:
A. 4 to 6 hours B. 6 to12 hours
C. 12 to 24 hours D. 2 to 3 days

76. Pus formation in a wound is seen mostly around:
A. 6 to 12 hours B. 12 to 24 hours
C. 36 to 48 hours D. 3 to 5 days

77. Bruise attains green discoloration by:
A. 1 day B. 2-3 days
C. 5-6 days D. 7-12 days

78. Bruise present on the following area does not show typical color changes:
A. Ear lobes B. Tongue
C. Conjunctiva D. Genitalia

79. Color changes in bruise start from:
A. Center of the bruise
B. Periphery of the bruise
C. Uniformly all over the bruise
D. Any area of the bruise

80. Rail track bruising results from:
A. Fall on railway track
B. Blow by a whip
C. Railway accident
D. Blow by an iron rod

---

72 D 73 D 74 C 75 C 76 C 77 C 78 C
79 B 80 B

81. Black gun powder contains:

A. Antimony sulphide
B. Pot nitrate
C. Pot chlorate
D. Mercury fulminate

82. Smokeless gun powder may contain following *except:*

A. Nitro cellulose
B. Nitro glycerine
C. Nitro benzene
D. Nitro guanidine

83. Rifled firearms include following *except:*

A. Revolvers **B.** Pistols
C. Shot guns **D.** Machine guns

84. Secondary markings on the fired bullet are:

A. Called class characteristics
B. Produced by toothed forceps while removing
C. Called individual characteristics
D. Produced due to manufacturing defects

85. Paradox gun is:

A. Smooth bore gun with rifling at muzzle end
B. Smooth bore gun with rifling at breach end
C. Smooth bore gun with narrowing at the muzzle end
D. Anti clockwise rifling grooves

86. Singeing of hair at the entrance wound of shot gun may be seen upto the distance of:

A. 15 cm **B.** 30 cm
C. 45 cm **D.** 60 cm

87. Large central hole with some pellet holes at the periphery may be seen in case shot gun is fired from the distance of:

A. 0.5 meter **B.** 0.5 to 1 meter
C. 2-3 meters **D.** 4-5 meters

81 B 82 C 83 C 84 C 85 A 86 A 87 C

88. Contact entrance wound caused by a revolver on the head show:
- **A.** Singeing of hair around the wound
- **B.** Blackening around the wound
- **C.** Tattooing around the wound
- **D.** Cruciate splitting of the wound

89. Depth of stab wound is:
- **A.** Equal to the length of blade
- **B.** More than the length of blade
- **C.** Less than the length of blade
- **D.** Not related with the length of blade

90. Spread of bullets in cm is equal to approximately:
- **A.** Half the distance of fire in meters
- **B.** Same distance of fire in meters
- **C.** 2 and half times the distance of fire in meters
- **D.** 5 times the distance of fire in meter

91. Arborescent marking are seen in burns due to:
- **A.** Electricity
- **B.** Phosphorus
- **C.** Lightning
- **D.** U.V. rays

88 D 89 D 90 C 91 C

4

Violent Asphyxial Deaths

Violent Asphyxial Deaths

Triad of Asphyxia

- Cyanosis (plum colour)
- Petechiae (Tardieu's Spots*)
- Visceral Congestion

Hanging	**Strangulation**	**Suffocation**	**Drowning**
Typical	Throttling	Smothering	Wet Drowning
Atypical	Garroting	Traumatic Asphx.	Dry Drowning
Complete	Mugging	Burking	Delayed Drowning
Partial	Bansdola	Gagging	Hydrocution
Mostly Suicidal*	***Mostly Homicidal****	Café Coronary	
		Purest form of Asphyxia*	

Asphyxia in Greek, means **"Absence of pulsation"**, but in **Forensic** parlance it means **"Interference with oxygenation"**.

Gordon's Classification of ANOXIA (Lack of oxygen)
• **Anoxic Anoxia:** Oxygen from atmosphere cannot get entry into blood, e.g., Hanging, Strangulation, Smothering, Choking, Traumatic asphyxia etc.

Contd.

Contd.

- **Anaemic Anoxia:** Inability of blood to carry sufficient oxygen due to low haemoglobin contents.
- **Stagnant Anoxia:** Where the circulation of blood is impaired so that there is lack of oxygenated blood transport to the tissues.
- **Histotoxic Anoxia:** Oxygen although freely available in the bloodstream—cannot be utilized by the tissues.
  - (a) *Extracellular:* Tissue oxygen enzyme system is poisoned. Viz. Cyanide, in which the **cytochrome-oxidase system** is affected; Hypnotic; Anaesthetic drug; Aluminium phosphide poisoning.
  - (b) *Pericellular:* Oxygen cannot gain access to the cell because of the decrease in the **cell membrane permeability**. E.g., halogenated hydrocarbons–**Chloroform, Halothane, etc.**
  - (c) *Metabolite Histotoxic Hypoxia:* The end products of cellular respiration cannot be removed thereby preventing further metabolism. **E.g., Uraemia, CO_2 poisoning.**
  - (d) *Substrate:* Inadequate food for efficient metabolism by the cell.

STAGES OF ASPHYXIA

S-Q-C-A: Struggle - forceful breathing→ **Q**uiescence - unconscious, lifeless→**C**onvulsions - disturbs scene, incontinence→**A**pnea - lifeless, weak pulse.
[Stage of forced respiration - Stage of convulsions - Stage of paralysis]

Histology of Asphyxia

- Disruption of alveolar septa with Haemorrhage in alveoli and oedema.
- Brick red discoloration of nerve cells in Cortex.
- Pallor and Vacuolar degeneration – Purkinje cells, Hepatocytes.
- Chemical marker – **Hypoxanthine** in blood and vitreous.

Hanging

Complete Hanging

- Hanging is that form of asphyxia which is caused by suspension of the body by a ligature, which encircles the neck, **the constricting force* being the weight of the body.**

Partial Hanging

- The bodies are partially suspended; the weight of the head (5-6 kg) acts as the constricting force.

Typical Hanging

- In typical hanging, the ligature runs from the midline above the thyroid cartilage symmetrically upward on both sides of the neck to the occipital region.

Atypical Hanging

When the knot is placed at site other than that seen in typical hanging.

Type of Knots

1. **Fixed knot:**
   - Most common pattern.
   - Ligature mark seen is 'inverted V shape'.
2. A **running noose:** Ligature mark is horizontal.

Causes of Death

1. Asphyxia.
2. Venous congestion.
3. Combined asphyxia and venous congestion is the most common cause of death.
4. Cerebral anemia.
5. Reflex vagal inhibition.
6. Fracture or dislocation of the cervical vertebrae.

Pressure Required for Closure of Neck Structures

Structure	*Pressure (Kg)*
Jugular Vein	2
Carotid Artery	5
Trachea	15
Vertebral Artery	30

Tardieu's Spots (also known as Bayard's Ecchymoses)

- These are Ecchymoses.
- Caused due to acute rise in ***Venous Pressure.***
- Rarely seen in Parietal Pleura or Peritoneum except Bleeding Diathesis.
- Present above the level of obstruction, where capillaries are least supported, e.g., Face, conjunctiva, epiglottis
- **Tardieu's spots** can be as a result of intense lividity, leading to postmortem rupture of dependently engorged blood vessels unrelated to asphyxia or any other mechanism of death (non-specific).
- Rarely seen in plastic bag suffocation, atmospheric suffocation.

Amussat's Sign*: A transverse (horizontal) laceration of the intimal layer of carotid arteries in Hanging also known as ***Ladder Tear*** (also seen in Vehicular Accidents). It is due to combination of:
(a) **Radial Force**–ligature material.
(b) **Axial Traction**–weight of suspended body.

Fatality

- The usual period is 3 to 5 minutes.
- Fatal hypoxia takes place when $\mathbf{O_2}$ level fall below **20%** of normal.

Postmortem Appearance

External Features

- **The ligature mark** in the neck is the most important and specific sign of death from hanging. The ligature mark is situated above the level of thyroid cartilage between the larynx and the chin in 80 percent cases, it is obliquely placed; does not completely encircles the neck.
- Face is congested, puffed up and bluish.
- The eyes are frequently protruded and the conjunctiva congested the pupils are usually dilated.
- Tongue is protruded and may be caught between the teeth.

- Dribbling of saliva from the angle of mouth is the *most important external sign of antemortem hanging*. *(OPPOSITE side to that of knot*).*
- **Le facies sympathique*:** It is a vital sign of **antemortem hanging*.**
  When the knot presses the cervical sympathetic trunk, the eye on that side remain open and the pupil is dilated.
- Seminal emission is common, in case of antemortem hanging.
- **In true suicidal hanging** the rope moves from above downwards.

Internal Features

Fracture Hyoid Bone

Abduction fracture or ***Anterior-Posterior Compression Fracture*** is seen in hanging:

- Hyoid bone is fractured in 15-20% cases. Are seen in persons above 40 years.
- Most common site of fracture of hyoid bone in hanging is at the **junction of the inner two third and outer third of greater cornu** (cf. ***Inward compression fracture*** or Adduction fracture seen in case of throttling).

Judicial Hanging

- Legal death sentence is carried out by hanging the criminal in India.
- The cause of death in judicial is (**Brainstem Damage**).
- ***The knot is placed below chin (most efficient method)***,* the length of rope from the point of suspension is equal to the height of individual. There is a sudden drop, resulting in fracture and dislocation of Upper Cervical Vertebrae (Fracture **of C2 from C3,** rarely C3 and C4).

Strangulation

- Strangulation is that form of asphyxia which is caused from constriction of the neck by a ligature without suspending the body.

- The mark in strangulation completely encircles the neck transversely, below the thyroid cartilage.
- During a postmortem on a suspected case of strangulation in situ examination of neck structures is done before opening the skull and the chest.
- Most important sign of strangulation is ligature mark.
- Fracture of thyroid cartilage is more common in strangulation by ligature.
  - **Mugging**—Homicidal strangulation, by holding the neck in the bend of elbow.
  - **Bansdola**—Strangulation with sticks (Homicidal strangulation).
  - **Garroting**—Strangulation by twisting a lever like a tourniquet, homicidal strangulation.

Traditionally practiced in **'SPAIN'** as a mode of execution.

Throttling

1. Manual strangulation (always homicidal).
2. Fracture of the hyoid bone in 30-50% cases
   – In Hyoid there is ***inward compression fracture**** (Adduction #).
   – The periosteum is torn on the outer side.
3. Fracture of the thyroid cartilage and of hyoid bone are usually found in above 40 years.

Signs of Asphyxia

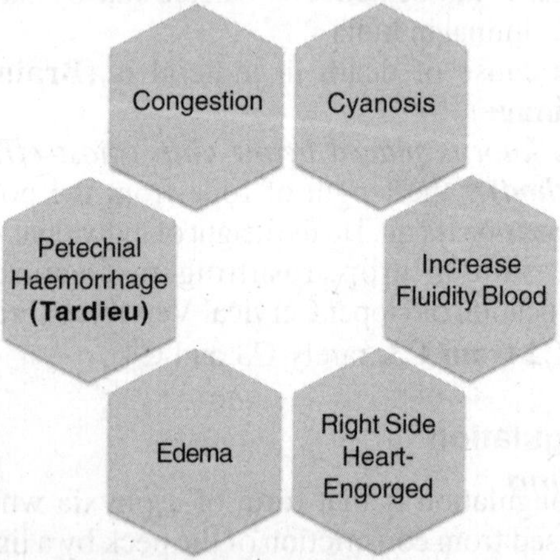

Diagnostic Hexagon of Asphyxia

- Intense congestion and deep cyanosis of the head and neck is seen in strangulation.
- The eyes wide open and pupils dilated.
- The tongue swollen and protruded.
- Petechial haemorrhages are common into the skin of the eyelids, face, forehead, behind the ears and scalp.
- Blood stained froth may escape from the mouth and nostrils and there may be bleeding from nose and ears.
- There is severe congestion and haemorrhage into the subcutaneous tissue in and above the area compressed.
- The intima of the carotid artery is not usually damaged.
- Fracture of the thyroid cartilage is more common.

Simon's hemorrhages: Ventral intervertebral hemorrhages under the **(ALL) Anterior Longitudinal Ligament** may be seen in Hanging. Most common site – lumbar region of the spine.

Types of Suffocation

Smothering

Death due to mechanical occlusion of the mouth and nose that prevents breathing.

Overlaying

It is a type of smothering. Overlaying or compression suffocation results due to compression of the chest, so as to prevent breathing.

Burking

- It is a method of homicidal smothering and traumatic asphyxia.
- William Burk and William Hare killed 16 persons in Edinburg using bunking.

Gagging

It's a type of asphyxia in which a cloth is forced into the mouth.

Cafe Coronary (Food Asphyxia) is a type of Accidental Choking:

- The term, 'Cafe Coronary', was coined by **Dr Roger Haugen.**
- The victim may be observed slumping over the dining table or collapsing suddenly while walking across the room after having meals, with **no signs of respiratory distress.**
- The original series of deaths involved well-nourished businessmen dying suddenly and unexpectedly in restaurants and cafes, while sitting or shortly after sitting in their chairs, **as if (appears to be) they died of heart attack. Hence the name, 'cafe coronary' (Misnomer).**
- **Cause of Death is Choking*–Vasovagal Syncope/Laryngeal Spasm–Secondary Cardiac Arrest (not Primary Cardiac Arrest or Heart Attack).**
- However, autopsy usually revealed a bolus of food in the pharynx or larynx.
- The suppression of gag-reflex due to alcohol or drugs makes the individual susceptible to Cafe Coronary.
- **Heimlich Maneuver** can prevent choking and Cafe Coronary.

Traumatic Asphyxia

- **First described by Ollivier in Paris Stampede Case (1837) by using a term *MASQUE ECCHYMOTIQUE****, which consisted of cranio-cervical cyanosis, subconjunctival haemorrhage, and cerebral vascular engorgement.

  The Snake **Boa constrictor** kills by causing Traumatic Asphyxia.
- Traumatic asphyxia results from respiratory arrest due to *mechanical fixation of the chest**, so that the normal movement of the chest wall are prevented.
- Common cause is crushing by falls of earth in a coal mine or during tunelling or in a building collapse.

- An intense cyanosis of deep purple or purple red colour of the head, neck and upper chest, above the level of compression is the prominent feature.

Sexual Asphyxia

- Partial asphyxia causes cerebral disturbance with feeling of sexual gratification.
- These cases are associated with some form of abnormal sexual behaviour, usually ***masochism and transvestism:***
  - **Kotzwarraism***→Term associated with auto eroticism.
- Death is mostly accidental.

DROWNING

- **Definition:** Drowning is suffocation due to immersion of the nostrils and mouth in a liquid. *(Chullu Bhurr Pani—**a common Hindi idiom also**—can lead to drowning).*

Phases of Drowning

Breath holds→ Inhalation of water, coughing, vomiting and loss of consciousness→ Convulsions, respiratory arrest then cardiac arrest.

Brouardel's Experiment on Stages of Drowning

i. Stage of surprise (5-10 seconds).
ii. First stage of respiratory arrest (1 min).
iii. Stage of deep respiration (1 min).
iv. Second stage of respiratory arrest (1 min).
v. Stage of terminal gasp (30 seconds).

Types of Drowning

A. Typical Drowning

1. **Wet Drowning (Primary Drowning)**
   - The water is inhaled into lungs.
   - The cause of death is cardiac arrest/asystole confusion killer.
     (Sea Water→**C**ardia-**C**-water) or ventricular **F**ibrillation, **F**resh Water.

B. Atypical Drowning

1. "Dry Drowning"

a. *Vagal inhibition (cardiac arrest, laryngeal shock):* Loss of consciousness is usually instantaneous.

b. *Laryngeal spasm:* There is no evidence of aspiration of liquid and there are the typical signs of an asphyxial death including facial cyanosis and petechial haemorrhages.

Circumstances common to these deaths are:

a. Entering the water feet first.
b. Surprise or unpreparedness.
c. A state of hypersensitivity, viz. alcohol intoxication.
d. "Duck-diving" or any clumsy diving with abdominal impact against the water can produce a similar result.
There may be instantaneous rigor (cadaveric spasm).

2. Secondary Drowning ("secondary drowning", post-immersion syndrome)

- It is also called delayed drowning.
- The individual who is resuscitated, survives for 1 day but develop complications like:
  - Electrolyte imbalance.
  - Metabolic acidosis etc.
- Signs of asphyxia absent.
- Delayed death.

3. Immersion Syndrome:

- Hydrocution due to cold water.
- *Submersion* syndrome.
- The cause of death is vagal inhibition due to:
  a. Cold water.
  b. Water striking epigastrium.

Causes of Death

- Asphyxia.
- Ventricular fibrillation.
- Laryngeal spasm.
- Vagal inhibition.
- Exhaustion.
- Injuries.

Phases of Drowning

Submersion→Struggle→Exhaustion→Drowning begins→Breath holding till CO_2 accumulation→ Respiration stimulation→Inhalation of water→Gulping →Coughing and vomiting→Loss of consciousness.

Fatal Period

- Death is almost invariable when the period of submersion **exceeds 10 minutes.**
- The survival rate from potentially fatal salt water submersion is about 80% whereas in fresh water it is less than 50%.
- **Hyperventilation** before drowning can cause rapid death, as CO_2 will be flushed out and there will be **no hypercapnia,** which is necessary to stimulate respiratory centre.

  Hyperventilation artificially depletes CO_2 causing a low blood carbon dioxide condition called hypocapnia. Hypocapnia reduces the reflexive respiratory drive, allows the delay of breathing and leaves the diver susceptible to loss of consciousness from hypoxia, thereby decreasing 'mortality time'.

Postmortem Appearance

- Atypical arrest due to drowning, cardiac arrest due to drowning, laryngospasm and drowning in unconscious state.
- **Postmortem staining**
  1. In stagnant water postmortem staining is present is usually found on the face, the upper part of chest, hands, lower arms, feet.
  2. If the body is moving during drowning, postmortem staining does not appear.
- Petechial haemorrhages are seen in subpleural tissues of lungs.
- **Froth in drowning**
  - A **fine, white, lathery, tenacious, persistent, and copious froth** is seen at mouth and nostrils—most characteristic external sign of drowning.

- Absence of foam in drowning can be found in death due to laryngeal spasm and immersion syndrome.
- Regurgitation of gastric contents into the larynx and trachea in cases of drowning is due to vomit reflex due to medullary hypoxia.
- *Froth without mucous* is seen in death due to:
  - Strangulation.
  - Acute pulmonary edema.
  - Electrical shock.
  - During an epileptic fit.
  - In opium poisoning.
  - Putrefaction.

- **Washer Woman's Hand:** Wrinkling of limbs indicate that body was in water. The skin becomes sodden, thickened, wrinkled and white in color within **12-18 hours.** Bleaching of the cuticle becomes quite evident after **12 hours** of immersion.
- **Cutis Anserina** (goose skin or goose flesh) in which the skin has granular and puckered appearance may be seen. It proves that molecular death present at the time of drowning.
- **Cadaveric spasm:** Weeds, grass, sticks, leaves etc. floating in water may be firmly grasped in the hands due to cataleptic rigidity (surest sign of antemortem drowning).*
- **Emphysema aquosum** (also known as emphyseme hydroaerique)
  - In wet drowning lungs are over distended and alveolar walls are torn.
  - The pleural surface has a **marbled appearance with grey-blue to dark red areas** interspersed with pink and yellow-grey zones of more aerated tissue.
  - Contrary to popular belief lung weights in fresh water drowning are same as from lung weights in salt water drowning.
  - On section an edematous condition is seen.
- **Paltauf's haemorrhages:** The alveolar walls may rupture due to increased pressure during forced expiration and produce **subpleural haemorrhage**

with blurred margins known as **'Paltauf's haemorrhages'**.

- **Middle Ear and Mastoid Cell Haemorrhage: Bluish purple discoloration** of the bone of the roof of mastoid air cells may be seen.
- **Shoulder-Girdle Bruises: B**ruise or rupture muscles particularly those of the shoulder girdle, neck and chest (most often the scaleni and pectoralis major). Haemorrhages may be bilateral and tend to follow the lines of the muscle bundles.
- **Water in GIT**
  - Most important evidence for drowning— water in stomach **(Sign of Moro).**
  - Water can be absent in stomach in cases of drowning due to sudden death, due to vagal inhibition.
  - Presence of water in stomach in case of drowning 70% cases.
  - The small intestine may contain water in 20% cases.
  - This sign is regarded as *positive evidence of death by drowning* as it depends on peristaltic movement which is a vital act.
- **Temporal bone haemorrhages** is seen in:
  - Drowning
  - Hanging
  - Head injury
  - CO poisoning.
- **Gettler's Chloride Test** *(Historical Value – Some historical examiners still ask)*
  - To differentiate fresh water drowning from sea water drowning.
  - Gettler test is NOT absolute proof of drowning **and of no help (no longer used):**
    - After 12 hours of death following drowning.
    - Putrefaction.
    - Vagal inhibition or laryngeal spasm.
    - Patent foramen ovale.
    - Brackish water.
  - Fresh water drowning, chloride content of **the left side** of the heart is 50% **lower (FiLL)**.

Moritz's Magnesium Test

High levels of plasm magnesium in left heart blood when contrasted with right heart blood is considered to reflect absorption on Mg from the **salt water.**

Drowning in Fresh Water

- Death in fresh water drowning in comparison to salt water is earlier.
- Drowning in fresh water leads to hemolysis and hemodilution, hyponatraemia/**hyperkalemia** leading to sodium/potassium imbalance together with myocardial hypoxia resulted in a dramatic collapse of systolic pressure quickly followed in the majority of cases by ventricular **F(fresh)-ibrillation.**
- In **F**resh water drowning, chloride content of the **L**eft side of the heart is 50% **L**ower (Memorizer-**Fi-LL).**

  PQZ→

  "Hemolytical garland" is seen in fresh water drowning.

  Razkazov-Lukomsky-Paltauf macules more often in fresh water submersion (73.07%) compared to that after sea water (35.66%).

Drowning in Sea Water (Cardia-C-water)

- Due to high salinity of sea water (usually over 3% NaCl), water is drawn from blood into lung tissue, and produces severe pulmonary oedema and **hypernatraemia,** increase in magnesium ion.
- The pulse pressure decreases slowly then A-V dissociation but not ventricular fibrillation. Half of the water content of the circulating blood is absorbed into the alveoli. This causes haemo-concentration, the cause of death is **Bradycardia – Cardiac Asystole*.**
- In sea water drowning, chloride content of the left side of the heart is higher **(Gettler's Test)***.

Diatoms (Bacillariophyceae)

- Diatoms are microscopic, unicellular, **silica** coated algae, coated algae.
- The bone marrow of **femur,** has maximum concentration of diatoms (**Ideal bone**).
- Most commonly used bone is **sternum.**
- Diatoms are examined by **acid digestion technique**.
- Presence of diatoms in bone marrow is the most important internal sign of antemortem drowning.
  - **In 1941 Incze** demonstrated that, during drowning, diatoms could enter the systemic circulation via the lungs.

Diagnosis

- The reliable signs of drowning at autopsy are:
  1. Antemortem drowning is **best demonstrated** by fine, white froth are the mouth and nose.
  2. The presence of weeds, stones etc. grasped in hand, show antemortem drowning due to cadaveric spasm.
  3. The presence of the fine froth at lungs and air passages.
  4. The voluminous water-loaded lungs.
  5. The presence of water in stomach and intestine.
  6. Finding of diatoms in the tissues.
- The above signs are not found if death occurs due to vagal inhibition.
- In the water the body floats face down with the head lower than the rest of the body so **that lividity is most prominent** on the head, neck and anterior chest. Also **Putrefaction begins first** within the areas of lividity, i.e., the head, neck and anterior chest.

  Postmortem cooling in water about twice as fast as in air and reaches the temperature of the water usually within 5 to 6 hours.
- The postmortem staining is not developed in drowning if the body is constantly moving, it is said ***"Rolling body gathers no postmortem hypostasis!!"***.

SPECIFIC SIGNS OF SINKING
• **Krushevsky's Sign:** Respiratory tracts full of **small foamy white bubbles.** • **Rasskazov-Lukomsky's Spots:** Reddening Edema of mucosa of respiratory tracts, increasing emphysema of lungs, pale and dim hemorrhages on lung surface. • **Sign of Moro:** Presence of water in a **small intestine and abdominal cavity.** • **Sabinsky-Orahovatz sign:** The **Spleen** becomes anaemic. • **Sign of Sveshnikov:** Presence of liquid of drowning environment in the **Sphenoid Sinus.** • Increase in of liver size and presence of Plankton in inner organs.

MCQs

1. Most reliable sign of antemortem hanging is:
- **A.** Congested face
- **B.** Protruded tongue
- **C.** Hard and pale ligature mark
- **D.** Dribbling of saliva

2. In judicial hanging fracture dislocation of cervical vertebrae occur between:
- **A.** C_1 and C_2
- **B.** Base of skull and C_1
- **C.** C_2 and C_3
- **D.** C_5 and C_6

3. Ligature mark of hanging is:
- **A.** Transversely placed
- **B.** At the level of thyroid cartilage
- **C.** Completely encircles the neck
- **D.** Hard, pale and parchment like

4. Adduction fracture of hyoid bone may be seen in:
- **A.** Ligature strangulation
- **B.** Manual strangulation
- **C.** Hanging
- **D.** Bansdola strangulation

5. Atypical hanging means:
- **A.** Body is completely suspended
- **B.** Some part of the body resting on an object
- **C.** Knot present on the back of head
- **D.** Knot present near the right ear

1 D **2** C **3** D **4** B **5** D

6. **Transverse tear in the intima of carotid arteries may be seen in:**
   A. Partial hanging
   B. Judicial hanging
   C. Bansdola strangulation
   D. Garroting

7. **A type of homicidal strangulation is:**
   A. Lynching B. Smothering
   C. Burking D. Garroting

8. **For diatoms test the best site for taking sample is:**
   A. Lungs
   B. Bone marrow in ulna
   C. Bone marrow in femur
   D. Muscle

9. **About 2 kgms of pressure on the neck can occlude:**
   A. Carotid arteries B. Vertebral arteries
   C. Trachea D. Jugular veins

10. **Death in sexual asphyxia is normally:**
    A. Homicidal B. Suicidal
    C. Accidental D. Judicial

11. **The cause of death in cafe-coronary is:**
    A. Laryngeal spasm
    B. Coronary insufficiency
    C. Coronary thrombosis
    D. Myocardial ischaemia

12. **Death is mostly accidental in:**
    A. Traumatic asphyxia B. Hanging
    C. Strangulation D. Smothering

13. **Cause of death in fresh water drowning is:**
    A. Myocardial ischaemia
    B. Laryngeal spasm
    C. Vagal inhibition
    D. Ventricular fibrillation

---

6 B 7 D 8 C 9 D 10 C 11 A 12 A
13 D

14. **Cause of death in hydrocution is:**
    A. Asphyxia
    B. Cardiac arrest
    C. Pulmonary edema
    D. Electrolyte disturbance

15. **Hyperkalemia is normally associated with:**
    A. Dry drowning
    B. Fresh water drowning
    C. Sea water drowning
    D. Hydrocution

16. **Death in dry drowning is due to:**
    A. Laryngeal spasm
    B. Vagal inhibition of heart
    C. Hyperkalemia
    D. Exhaustion

17. **Hypostasis on the head and face, hands and feet are seen in death from:**
    A. Hanging
    B. Strangulation
    C. Traumatic asphyxia
    D. Drowning (in moving water no hypostasis)

18. **Which of the following is an important sign of antemortem drowning?**
    A. Washerwoman's hands and feet
    B. Cutis anserina
    C. Weeds held infirmly hands
    D. Petecheal haemorrhages in the eyes

19. **Paltauf's haemorrhages are seen in:**
    A. Eyes B. Lungs
    C. Heart D. Mesentery

20. **Commonly tissue preserved for the detection of diatoms in drowning death is:**
    A. Lungs B. Stomach
    C. Liver D. Sternum

21. **Hyperventilation drowning deaths are:**
    A. Accidental B. Suicidal
    C. Homicidal D. None of the above

---

14 B 15 B 16 A 17 D 18 C 19 B 20 D
21 A

22. Burking consists of:
A. Smothering and traumatic asphyxia
B. Choking and drowning
C. Gagging only
D. Traumatic asphyxia only

23. The conclusive postmortem finding of death by drowning:
A. Cutis anserina
B. Presence of water in the middle ear
C. Edematous lungs
D. Demonstration of diatoms in the organs of the body

24. White lathery froth is seen in deaths due to:
A. Drowning
B. Hanging
C. Organophosphorus poisoning
D. Mineral acid poisoning

25. Fractures of the hyoid bone results from all *except:*
A. Throttling
B. Hanging
C. Choking
D. Ligature strangulation

26. Death of judicial hanging is because of:
A. Vasovagal shock
B. Occlusion of airway
C. Fracture dislocation of upper cervical vertebra
D. Coma

27. Which of the following is seen very rarely in hanging?
A. Fracture of hyoid cartilage
B. Fracture of thyroid cartilage
C. Staining of saliva
D. Ligature mark

---

22 A 23 D 24 A 25 C 26 C 27 A,C,D

28. Hanging with the feet touching the ground is seen in:

A. Partial hanging
B. Complete hanging
C. Homicidal hanging
D. Suicidal hanging

29. Hyoid fracture is seen in:

A. Hanging **B.** Strangulation
C. Burking **D.** Throttling

30. Petechial haemorrhages in drowning is seen in:

A. Subpleural tissues of lung
B. Submucosa of trachea
C. Bronchioles
D. Alveoli

31. Paltauf's haemorrhage occurs in which injury?

A. Strangulation **B.** Hanging
C. Drowning **D.** Burns

32. Horizontal ligature mark in the neck is seen in:

A. Throttling
B. Hanging
C. Strangulation by ligature
D. Chocking

33. Emphysema aqueosum is seen in:

A. Wet drowning
B. Secondary drowning
C. Dry drowning
D. Immersion syndrome

34. Which of the following sign will indicate that the death was antemortem?

A. Cutis anserina
B. Washerwoman's skin
C. Weed and grass in the hands
D. Cyanosis

---

28 A 29 A,D 30A 31 C 32 C 33 A
34 C

35. Cafe coronary commonly occurs when a person is:

A. Intoxicated
B. Eating fatty food
C. Eating meat
D. Eating fish

36. Accidental drowning is ruled out if:

A. The body is tied up inside a gunny bag
B. Hand and feet are tied by a ligature in way that is inconsistent with suicidal drowning
C. Heavy weights are attached in such a way that suicidal drowning is excluded
D. All of the above

37. Froth of drowning can be differentiated from that due to other causes by:

A. Microscopic detection of mucous
B. Detecting excess of salt in the froth
C. Both A and B
D. None of the above

38. A method of homicidal smothering and traumatic asphyxia is known as:

A. Choking
B. Gagging
C. Burking
D. Overlying

39. Hyperventilation before drowning:

A. Can cause rapid death
B. Does not alter the process of drowning
C. Can cause delayed death
D. Can cause secondary drowning

40. Atypical arrest due to drowning is:

A. Cardiac arrest due to drowning
B. Laryngospasm due to drowning
C. Drowning in unconcious state
D. All of the above

35 A 36 D 37 A 38 C 39 A 40 D

41. Most common type of drowning is:
A. Suicidal
B. Accidental
C. Homicidal
D. All of the above

42. Le facies sympathique is seen in:*
A. Traffic accident
B. Hanging
C. Stragulation
D. Myocardial infarction

43. Suicidal drowning differs from homicidal drowning by the following *except:*
A. Absence of signs of struggle
B. Marks of violence on body absent
C. Untorn clothes
D. None of the above

44. Hanging is defined as:
A. Suspension of body by a ligature, body weight acting as constricting force
B. Suspension of body by ligature after death
C. Obliteration of air passages by external compression
D. Mechanical interference to respiration

45. Maximum congestion is seen in:
A. Choking
B. Hanging
C. Strangulation
D. Drowning

46. Oedema aquosum occurs in:
A. Submersion of unconscious
B. Dry drowning
C. Secondary drowning
D. Immersion syndrome

47. Getler's test is positive in:
A. Hanging
B. Poisoning
C. Strangulation
D. Drowning

41 B **42** B **43** D **44** A **45** C **46** A **47** D

48. Dry drowning is defined as:
- **A.** Drowning in sea water
- **B.** Drowning in cold water, death being due to cardiac arrest
- **C.** Drowning of a dehydrated body
- **D.** Drowning where death is due to laryngospasm

49. The most specific feature of death due to hanging is:
- **A.** Tardieu spots
- **B.** Ligature mark
- **C.** Fracture of thyroid cartilage
- **D.** Dribbling of saliva

50. Extensive bruising of neck muscles of ecchymosis of subcutaneous tissues in neck is characteristic of:
- **A.** Hanging
- **B.** Strangulation
- **C.** Throttling
- **D.** Burking

51. One of the following is a definite sign of death due to drowning:
- **A.** Sand and mud in the mouth and nostrils
- **B.** Fine lathery froth in the mouth and nostrils
- **C.** Washerwoman's hands and feet
- **D.** Diatoms in bone marrow

52. In a case of hanging neck ligature marks are example of:
- **A.** Contusion
- **B.** Printed abrasion
- **C.** Laceration
- **D.** Bruise

53. Gettler's test is positive in:
- **A.** Hanging
- **B.** Poisoning
- **C.** Strangulation
- **D.** Drowning

---

48 D **49** D **50** C **51** D **52** B **53** D

54. The postmortem finding seen in smothering:
- **A.** Abrasion on the inner side of the upper lip
- **B.** Fracture body of hyoid
- **C.** Thyroid fracture
- **D.** Curved marks on the neck

55. Acid digestion test is used for:
- **A.** To detect food content in stomach
- **B.** To detect fibre content in food
- **C.** To detect diatoms in drowning
- **D.** To detect metal pieces from gun injury

56. Cafe coronary is due to:
- **A.** MI
- **B.** Laryngeal spasm
- **C.** Strangulation
- **D.** Drowning

57. Lynching is:
- **A.** Practised in North America
- **B.** Practised by white people on Negroes
- **C.** Hanging publicly on a tree
- **D.** All of the above

54 A 55 C 56 B 57 D

5

Medicolegal Aspects: Sexual Offences

A. NATURAL OFFENCES

It includes those offences which are committed in order of nature, i.e., by penetration of the vagina by the penis., E.g., **Rape, Adultery, Incest.**

B. UNNATURAL OFFENCES

1. **Tribadism or Lesbianism**–Female homosexuality.
2. **Bestiality**–Sexual intercourse with lower animal.
3. **Sin of Gomarrah**–Buccal coitus, coitus per OS.
4. **Sodomy or Buggery**–Anal intercourse with a male or female, only proof is semen in anus.
5. Rape can fall in the category of Unnatural Sexual offence (as per new law).

C. SEXUAL PERVERSIONS

(A→Z please add newer terms as you find them)

- **Bondage–**The combining of Sadism and Masochism.
- **Exhibitionism–**Punishable under Sec 294 IPC.

- **Fetichism**–Sexual satisfaction by contact with articles of opposite sex.
- **Frotteurism–Contact with other persons** to obtain sexual gratification.
- **Lust murder**–Murder serves as stimulus for sexual act.
- **Masochism**–Opposite to sadism.
- **Masturbation** (Onanism, ipsation)–Is the deliberate self-stimulation, which effects sexual arousal.
- **Necrophagia**–Necros = Corpse; phagia = to eat.
- **Necrophilia**–Sexual intercourse with dead body.
- **Sadism**–Sexual gratification by torturing or inflicting pain on someone.
- **Satyriasis**–Incessant sexual desire in males. **Nymphomania** in females.
- **Transvestism**–Trans = opposite, vesta = clothing or **Eonism*.**
- **Undinism (Urolangia)**–Sexual pleasure by witnessing the act of urination.
- **Voyeurism (Scoptophilia NEET)–Peeping Tom.** It is sexual enjoyment from watching. Can be persecuted under **Sec. 354C IPC and Sec. 509 IPC.**

D. OTHER SEX-LINKED OFFENCES

1. **Sexual harassment (Sec. 354-A IPC)** is defined as physical contact and advances involving unwelcome and explicit sexual overtures, or demanding sexual favours, showing pornography against her will or making sexually tainted remarks. The offence is cognizable and bailable.
2. Indecent assault.
3. Stalking.
4. Acid Attacks.
5. **Obscenity (Exhibitionism)**. IPC Sections 292–294.

CRIMINAL LAW (AMENDMENT) ACT, 2013 – SIMPLIFIED

Justice J.S. Verma Committee report led to the passing of the Criminal Law (Amendment) Act, 2013, which brought several significant changes to the IPC, 1860 and the CrPC, 1973.

1. Rape

A. Section 375—Rape

Rape Law (New Changes): Significant changes made to section 375. **The new section** is seen as an improvement, the old section recognised rape only as the insertion of the penis into the vagina (Key words **are highlighted**).

A man is said to commit **rape if he penetrates his own penis, or makes another man penetrate his penis, into the *vagina, mouth, urethra or anus* of a woman,** or penetrates any other object, manipulates her body to cause penetration, or applies his own mouth, or makes another man apply his mouth to the vagina, anus or urethra of a woman.

7 Modes: Such actions have to be committed in one of **seven modes:**

I. against her **will**,
II. without her **consent**,
III. with her consent which has been obtained through **threats**,
IV. by **posing** as her husband,
V. with her consent which was taken when she was **intoxicated** by alcohol or other substances,
VI. with/without consent when she is under **the age of 18 years**** *(Statutory Rape),*
VII. when she is **unable** to give her consent.

Marital rape, is an exception to section 375, provided that the wife is not under 15 years of age. Sexual intercourse by a man with his own wife is not rape, if she is above 15 years of age (**Sec. 375 IPC**).

- **Will v/s Consent:** An act done against the will of a person is always without consent, but every act done without consent is not always against the will of the person.
- **Doctrine of Adverse Inference:** When the victim states that she did not consent, the **presumption** is usually in her favour; the consent is adjudged from the circumstances in which the act occurred. This is called an **adverse inference**, and it had been included in the Indian Evidence Act, 1872 under **Section 114-A IEA***.
- **III, IV and V** come into play in those circumstances where the consent of the victim was taken, but the woman was *unable to give "true consent"*.
- When a woman has consented to sexual intercourse, but withdraws her consent during sex, it is RAPE if the man forcibly continues in his act.
- A woman of **18 years and above** can give valid consent for sexual intercourse.
- Rape can be committed even when there is inability to produce erection of penis.
- Experts have proved that **rape and pleasure can occur simultaneously**, and pleasure cannot be taken as a sign of consent from the victim.
- Rape on virgin cause tear at **posterolateral position** of hymen **(4/8 'O Clock or 5/7' O Clock)**.
- **Hymen in a child may be placed high up or deep seated and may escape rupture during intercourse. (*NEET Exam)**
- Under the law rape can only be committed by a man, in **France*** where even a female can be charged of rape. In India, there is **no age limit** under which a boy is considered physically incapable of committing rape.
- Medical proof of intercourse is **not** legal proof of rape.
- Rape is a **cognizable offence.**

B. Section 376—Punishment For Rape

Sec. 376 (1) IPC: A man committing rape is punished with rigorous imprisonment for a term ≥ 7 years which may extend to life imprisonment and fine.

Sec. 376 (2) IPC: Punishment is rigorous imprisonment for **≥10 years or life** imprisonment (remainder of natural life) and fine, if rape is committed on a woman under following circumstances:

a. By a police officer, member of armed forces, public servant, management or on the staff of jail, remand home, women's or children's institution or hospital while under custody.
b. By a relative, guardian, teacher or a person of trust or authority, or in a position of control or dominance over the woman.
c. During communal or sectarian violence.
d. When she is under 16 years of age, pregnant or incapable of giving consent.
e. Who is physically or mentally disable.
f. Repeatedly on the same woman.
g. Causes grievous injury, mutilate or disfigures or endangers her life during the act.

376 A to E

A. Causing Death/Persistent Vegetative State (≥ 20 years).
B. Husband having sexual intercourse with wife during separation.
C. Rape by person in authority (Custodial Rape).
D. Gang Rape (≥ 20 years).
   Women who is part of the gang can be charged with Rape*.
E. Repeat offender (could be death sentence).

Severity of Punishment

1. **7 years** at the least, and may extend up to life imprisonment.
2. **10 years:** Any man who is a police officer, medical officer, army personnel, jail officer, public

officer or public servant commits rape may be imprisoned for **at least** ten years.

3. **20 years: Gangrape** has been prescribed a punishment of at least 20 years.
4. **Death Penalty:** A punishment of life imprisonment, extending to death has been prescribed for situations where the rape concludes with the death of the victim, or the victim entering into a coma.

C. Section 326A—Acid Attacks

The Amendment has made special provisions for acid attacks.

Acid has been defined as any substance which has a **corrosive nature**; it may include bleach, bathroom and toilet acid, Harpic, etc.

Under 326A: A person who throws or administers acid on another person and causes damage or deformity is liable for an imprisonment that is not less than **ten years**, and may extend to life imprisonment.

Any fine that is collected under section 326A **is granted to the victim for medical expenses**.

D. Sec. 326B IPC—Attempted Acid Attack

An attempt to throw acid upon a person is met with imprisonment of **up to seven years**, but not less than five years for the attacker, under section 326B.

The harm that is stipulated under the section need not be external physical harm, but it may also include harm caused to internal organs, as they are covered by the term "administering acid".

For e.g., X throws a chemical at Y; the chemical does not harm Y's face but it causes her to be blinded in one eye; this is covered by section **326A.**

[**Sec. 100 IPC:** The right of **Private defence against an assault.** The Amendment has introduced a new category of private defence which includes an **acid attack** within its ambit.]

Sec. 354A: Sexual Harassment

Definition: A man who makes unwelcome sexual advances, forcefully shows pornography or demands/ requests sexual favours from a woman commits the offence of **sexual harassment *simpliciter*** under section 354A.

Punishment: This is punishable by imprisonment of up to three years.

Making sexually coloured remarks also amounts to sexual harassment, which is punishable by imprisonment for up to one year.

Sec. 354B IPC: If a man assaults a woman with the intent of removing her clothes or compelling her to be naked, he commits an offence under section 354B, which is punishable with imprisonment between **three and seven years.**

Sec. 354C: Voyeurism is the next category of sexual harassment. Voyeurism is the act of watching a person engaged in private activities.

If a man watches a woman engaged in private activities, when the woman does not expect anyone to be watching, he has committed the offence of voyeurism under **section 354C** and is liable to be imprisoned between one and three years for the first time, and between three and seven years for subsequent convictions.

Sec. 354D IPC: Stalking is the last offence in the category of sexual harassment. It means following a person and making or attempting to make contact for personal interaction, despite a clear disinterest being displayed by the other person. Stalking may be committed both physically and through electronic media.

If a man stalks a woman, he may be punished with imprisonment of up to three years for the first time, and five years for the subsequent convictions.

Other Sections Related to Rape Laws
• **Sec. 114A IEA**–Presumption as to absence of consent in certain prosecutions for rape. **CR. PC LINKED TO RAPE LAWS** • **Sec. 26(a) CrPC**–Rape case trial by woman judge. • **Sec. 53(1) CrPC**–Reasonable force to examine **Accused***. • **Sec. 53(2) CrPC–Victim** to be examined under supervision of female RMP. • **Section 164A CrPC**–The victim to be medically examined within 24 hours of the receipt of the information of the rape. Key word **WITHOUT DELAY.** • **Section 327(2) of CrPC** lays down that in rape cases the judicial proceedings "shall be conducted in camera". • **Sec. 357C CrPC**–*Treatment and Information to Police:* All hospitals treatment, free of cost, to the survivor/victim of rape or acid attack, and should immediately inform the police. **IPC LINKED TO RAPE LAWS** • **Sec. 90 IPC**–If victim is less than 12 years, Parents'/Guardian's consent to be taken. • **Sec. 166-B IPC:** Denial of treatment of such victims is punishable under with imprisonment upto 1 year and with/without fine. • **Sec. 228A IPC**–Punishment of revealing identity of victim. • **Obscenity (Exhibitionism)**. IPC Sections 292–294: **Police** can directly prosecute an individual under Sec. 294 IPC. **[NEET Exam]** • **IPC Section 354:** Criminal Force or Assault Intended to Outrage Modesty. • **IPC Section 509:** Word, Gesture or Act Intended to Outrage Modesty. • **IPC Section 370:** Trafficking.

Contd.

Contd.

- ***POCSO:*** The sexual exploitation of children is also penalised under the new legislation called **"Protection of Children from Sexual Offences Act, 2012".**

Adultery (Sec. 497 IPC Deals with Adultery)

- Offence against marriage.
- If proven, adultery is a valid ground for divorce and nullity of marriage.
- An aggrieved husband can charge another man with adultery.
- A woman cannot be charged with the offence of adultery.

(NB→ Section 498 IPC–Enticing or taking away or detaining with criminal intent a married woman.)

Incest: Incest is a sexual intercourse by a man with a woman, who is closely, related to him by blood, e.g., a daughter, grand daughter, sister, stepsister, aunt and mother.

- In India, incest as such is not an offence.

Types of Incests

a. Oedipus complex—Son and mother.
b. Electra complex—Daughter and father.
c. Pharoan complex—Brother and sister.

2. Unnatural Offences

Voluntary sexual intercourse **against the order of nature** with any man or woman or animal is an unnatural sex offence under **Sec. 377 IPC.**

1. **Sodomy**
   - Sodomy is anal intercourse between two males or between a male and female.
   - It is also called Buggery.
   - It is called **gerontophilia** when the passive agent is an adult and **paederasty**, when the passive agent is a young boy, who is known as **catamite.**

- A **paedophile** is an adult who repeatedly engages in sexual activities **with children** below the age of puberty.
- The consent of sodomy is of no value, as both partners are punishable.

2. **Buccal coitus (Coitus per os or sin of Gommorah):** The male organ is introduced into mouth, usually of a young child.
3. **Tribadism**
   - **Female homosexuality** is known as tribadism or lesbianism.
     - Active Agent – **Dyke/butch**.
     - Passive Agent – Femme.
   - Sexual gratification of a woman is obtained by another woman.
   - The practice is usually indulged in by women who are mental degenerates or who suffer from Nymphomania (Excessive sexual desire).
   - Lesbians who are jealous of one another, when rejected may commit homicide, suicide or both.
4. **Bestiality**
   - **Bestiality** is sexual intercourse by a human being with a lower animal.
   - Dogs and cats are common animals for female, usually the animal manipulates the genitalia with its mouth and actual coitus is very rare.

3. Sexual Perversions

- Sexual perversions are persistently indulged sexual acts in which complete satisfaction is sought and obtained without sexual intercourse.
  1. **Uranism:** Perversion of sexual instinct.
  2. **Sadism:** In sadism, sexual gratification is obtained or increased from acts of physical cruelty or causing of pain upon one's partner.
  3. **Masochism:** In Masochism, sexual gratification is obtained or increased by suffering pain and cruelty from one's partner.

4. **Bondage:** The combining of sadism and masochism is called Bondage.

4. Sexual Oralism

- It is the obtaining of sexual pleasure from the application of the mouth to the sexual organs.
- **Feliatio** is the oral stimulation or manipulation of the penis either by the female or male.
- **Cunnilingus** is the oral stimulation of the female genitalia.

5. Masturbation

- Ipsation or Onanism.
- Masturbation is an offence when practised openly, e.g., in telephone booth, lavatories etc.

Eunuches

Male prostitutes are called–**Eunuches.**

- **Castrated Eunuches**–Hijrahs.
- **Eunuches with intact genitalia**–Zenana.

Medical Examination in a Rape Case (Please study a standard textbook at least once on this)

Potential Q Zone

Victim

- **Sec. 164-A(7) Cr. PC**–The court or the police have no power to compel victim for medicolegal examination against her will.
- Examination under Filtered UV light may detect semen or foreign debris on the skin.
- **SAFE kit:** Medical Kit for gathering and preserving physical evidence following an allegation of sexual assault. SAFE – Sexual Assault Forensic Evidence kit or Physical Evidence Recovery Kit (PERK). **Vitullo kit:** Medical kit

developed by Louis Vitullo to examine victim of sexual offence.

- Illuminated **Glaister-keen globe** can be used to stretch the hymen around for examination of the edges and gradation of tears.
- **Toluidine Blue Dye (TBD) helps in detection of microtrauma in sexual assault** – The most important benefit from TBD is the ability to identify **recent microtrauma** caused by blunt force trauma to the genitalia, sometimes using **COLPOSCOPE*** (for magnification).

Accused

- **Lugol's Iodine Test: Iodine solution** painted on the glans would reveal the presence of **vaginal epithelial cells**, turn **brown** due to the **glycogen**.

Seminal Fluid

Seminal fluid is a complex mixture of secretions from at least four male urogenital glands.

- The seminal vesicle gland – 60% to this mixture.
- Prostate gland contributes – 30%.
- Epididymis and bulbourethral glands account – 10%.
  - An average male ejaculate measures around 3.5 milliliters.
  - Each milliliter can contain between 10 and 50 million sperm cells.
  - Vasectomy, renders the male incapable of producing sperm somewhere between 2-4 months following that procedure.
  - Vasectomized, oligospermic, and aspermic males can produce normal amounts of seminal fluid.
  - Seminal stains have to be detected in cases of rape or attempted rape, sexual murder of the female, sodomy and bestiality.

  - Fertility of fluid has to be proved in disputed paternity.
  - Seminal fluid choline is originated from Leydig cells.
  - **Smegma:** If the smegma is present around glans of penis, it is suggestive of the fact that an individual did not have sexual intercourse in last 24 hours.
- Sperms make up 10–25% of the volume of the semen.
- Sperm density ranges from 60 to 100 million per ml.

CHEMICAL EXAMINATION

Confirmatory Tests for Semen

A. ***The Christmas Tree Stain:*** The most reliable confirmation for the presence of semen is the positive visual identification of sperm cells (or spermatozoa) using the Christmas tree stain. Two main reagents are used consecutively to produce this distinctive stain:
   - **Picroindigocarmine stains** the neck and **tail portions** of the sperm in green and **blue.**
   - **Nuclear Fast Red** (also known as **Kernechtrot**) gives the sperm heads a **red color** and the tips of the heads, an area known as acrosomal cap, a pink color.

B. ***RSID-Semen Strip Test:*** The **R**apid **S**tain **ID**entification-Semen test provides sensitivity as well as specificity to human semen. Similar in format to a pregnancy test strip, the RSID-semen test identifies the presence of the **seminal vesicle-specific antigen, or semenogelin.**

C. ***Prostate Specific Antigen:*** Another confirmatory test for semen is the detection of prostate specific antigen (PSA). Forensic labs utilize a **Glycoprotein P30 test** to screen for PSA. This test has replaced the quantitative analysis for acid phosphatase.

D. MHS-S1 is also positive and a highly reliable test for semen.

E. Lactate Dehydrogenase (LDH) Isoenzyme using Electrophoresis Method (**Absolute proof** of Semen) (Absolute proof of **sexual intercourse** is finding at least 1 unbroken sperm or LHD isoenzyme detection of sperm).

Motility of Sperm

- 100% sperms are motile till 3 hours.
- 50% sperms are motile till 8 hours.
- 10% sperms are motile till 24 hours.

Spermatozoa in wet mount is suggestive of intercourse within 24 hours*.

Presumptive Tests for Semen

A. Visual Detection: **Dried semen** can be visualized using blue light, **ultraviolet light** (also known as Wood's Lamp), semen will fluorescence due to the presence of molecules such as Flavin and choline-conjugated proteins. The color of this fluorescence will vary from blue to yellow, depending on the light equipment used.

B. The Acid Phosphatase Test (Walker Test)

- The prostatic secretion element of seminal fluid contains a very much **higher** percentage of Acid Phosphatase (AP).
- **Brentamine spot test:** In the presence of **Alpha-Naphthyl acid phosphate** and **Brentamine Fast Blue**, AP will produce a dark purple color in less than a minute.
- Analyses of post-coital vaginal swabs show that AP activity will markedly decrease after 24 hours and diminish after 48 hours.

Classical Tests

A. Florence Test (Choline Per. Iodide Crystals):

- The stain is extracted by 1% hydrochloric acid and a drop is placed on a glass slide.

- A drop of Florence solution (Postassium iodine, iodine and water) is allowed to run under the cover slip.
- If semen is present, dark-brown crystals of **choline iodide** appear immediately.
- They are rhombic crystals like haemin.
- **A negative test means the fluid is not semen.**

B. Barberio's Test:

- A saturated aqueous or alcoholic solution of **picric acid*** when added to spermatic fluid, produces yellow needle shaped rhombic crystals of spermine picrate.
- In **Barberio's test,** presence of **spermine in semen** is detected.
- Spermine picrate crystals are seen.

C. Creatine Phosphokinase: Level of CPK is high in seminal fluids, can be detected in old stains of 6 months.

D. Ammonium Molybdate Test:

- For semen stains, detect presence of phosphorous.

E. Serological typing of the semen is possible by **precipitin method.**

Fluorescence: Various naturally occurring chemicals present in body fluids such as semen, as well as latent fingerprints, may fluoresce under appropriate lighting conditions. Fluorescent body secretions include ***semen, saliva*** and ***sweat*** *(perspiration)*. Constituents of significance to the forensic scientist include various **fluorescent enzymes** and **proteins** contained in body fluids.

Phadebas Test: Saliva can be detected by l-amylase test.

MCQs

1. **Confirmatory sign of pregnancy is:**
   - **A.** Hegar's sign
   - **B.** Jacquemoers sign
   - **C.** Quickening
   - **D.** Foetal heart sounds

2. **Foetal heart sounds can be heard from:**
   - **A.** 3rd month onwards
   - **B.** 4th month onwards
   - **C.** 5th month onwards
   - **D.** 6th month onwards

3. **Maximum level of HCG in normal pregnancy is seen at about:**
   - **A.** 30 days after last menstrual period
   - **B.** 60 days after last menstrual period
   - **C.** 90 days after last menstrual period
   - **D.** 120 days after last menstrual period

4. **Superfoetation means:**
   - **A.** Fertilization of two ova of same menstrual cycle by two different acts of coitus
   - **B.** Uniovular twin pregnancy
   - **C.** Fertilization of a second ovum in already pregnant woman
   - **D.** Fertilization of two ovum with single act of coitus

5. **Posthumous child means:**
   - **A.** A child born after death of its father
   - **B.** A child born after death of its mother
   - **C.** A child born after artificial insemination
   - **D.** A child born after full term

1 D 2 C 3 B 4 C 5 A

6. **Immediately after delivery the uterus is felt at:**
   A. Mid point between umbilicus and xiphisternum
   B. Just below the umbilicus
   C. Mid point between umbilicus and pubic symphysis
   D. Just above pubic symphysis

7. **Uterus becomes a pelvic organ after delivery in about:**
   A. 1 week
   B. 2 weeks
   C. 3 weeks
   D. 4 weeks

8. **Valid consent by a female for sexual act can be given above the age of:**
   A. 12 years
   B. 15 years
   C. 16 years
   D. 18 years

9. **A female victim of sexual assault can give consent for medical examination only if she is above:**
   A. 12 years
   B. 16 years
   C. 18 years
   D. 21 years

10. **In a rape on small child the hymen:**
    A. Rupture, because it is very thin
    B. Rupture, because it is situated superficially
    C. Don't rupture because it is thick
    D. Don't rupture because it is situated deeply

11. **Triabadism means:**
    A. Sexual act by a female with another female
    B. Anal intercourse by a man with a female
    C. Anal intercourse by a man with a man
    D. Sexual act by a female with an animal

6 B 7 B 8 D 9 A 10 D 11 A

12. Transvestitism (Eonism) means:

A. Wearing clothes of opposite sex to attract attention

B. Wearing clothes of opposite sex to be associated with opposite sex

C. Wearing clothes of opposite sex to get sexual gratification

D. Wearing clothes of opposite sex in case

13. In I.P.C. unnatural sexual offences comes under:

A. Section 375
B. Section 376(A)
C. Section 376(B)
D. Section 377

14. In a male suffering from aspermia, the most suitable test for seminal stain is:

A. Florence test

B. Barberio test

C. Takayama test

D. Acid phosphatase test

15. Mobile sperm normally can be detected in vaginal aspirate after coitus upto:

A. 6 hours
B. 9 hours
C. 12 hours
D. 18 hours

16. Catamite refers to:

A. Active agent in sodomy

B. Any passive agent in sodomy

C. Small child acting as passive agent in sodomy

D. A female acting as passive agent in sodomy

17. Presence of smegma on the glans indicate:

A. Male has done sexual act recently

B. Male has not done sexual act in last 24 hours

C. Male has not done sexual act in last 48 hours

D. Male has not done sexual act in the last one week

18. In which of the following, legal action against the offender can be directly taken by police?

A. Incest
B. Fetichism
C. Exhibitionism
D. Sadism

---

12 C **13** D **14** D **15** D **16** C **17** B **18** C

19. Bestiality is:
A. Having intercourse with an animal
B. Cruelty to animals
C. Cruelty to fellow human
D. Beast like behaviour of an insane

20. Best test for seminal stains is:
A. Acid phosphatase test
B. Precipitin test
C. Florence test
D. Alkaline phosphatase test

21. Florence test detects:
A. Bilirubin
B. Urine
C. Semen
D. Blood

22. Barberio's test is done for:
A. Blood
B. Urine
C. Saliva
D. Semen

23. Paedophile is having anal intercourse with:
A. Older women
B. Children
C. Homosexual adult
D. Hijra

24. Acid phosphatase test is used for analysing:
A. Semen
B. Blood
C. Urine
D. Bile

25. All are tests for seminal stains *except:*
A. Takayama test
B. Barberio's test
C. Florence test
D. Acid phosphatase test

26. Of the following which does not categorize under rape? Sexual intercourse with:
A. Wife below 15 years
B. Wife above 20 years
C. Woman below 16 years
D. Woman above 20 years

19 A 20 A 21 C 22 D 23 B 24 A 25 A
26 B

27. Sexual perversions include:
- **A.** Masturbation
- **B.** Transvestism
- **C.** Fetichism
- **D.** All of the above

28. One of the following is a sure sign of rape:
- **A.** Ruptured hymen in a girl aged 20 years
- **B.** Presence of semen in the posterior fornix in a girl age 20 years
- **C.** Presence of semen in the posterior fornix in a girl aged 14 years
- **D.** Presence of semen in the posterior fornix in a married girl aged 16 years

29. The type of paraphilia where sexual excitement is obtained by wearing clothes of opposite sex is:
- **A.** Tribadism
- **B.** Voyeurism
- **C.** Transvestite
- **D.** Exhibitionism

30. Eonism is:
- **A.** Desire to identify with the opposite sex
- **B.** Intercourse with a lower animal
- **C.** Female homosexualism
- **D.** Oral sex
- **E.** Obtaining sexual gratification by seeing naked bodies

27 D 28 C 29 C 30 A

6

Infanticide is Murder

- The term, infanticide, comes from the Latin *infans, meaning unable to speak.*
  – It means the unlawful destruction of a child under the age of one year.
- **A stillborn** child is one which born after **28 weeks of pregnancy** and which did not breathe or show signs of life.
- **Fillicide*:** Killing of the child by its parents is called fillicide.
- **Neonaticide:** Killing of a child within 24 hours of birth.

I. DEAD BIRTH

- Most common cause of infant mortality rate is **prematurity.**
- A dead born child is one, which had died in uterus and shows one of the following signs after it is completely born.

  A. Rigor mortis at delivery.

  B. Maceration–Maceration is a process of **Aseptic Autolysis*** in dead born. The fetus surrounded by liquor amini for 3-4 days but no air*.
  - Child should remain in uterus for 24 hours in order to show signs of maceration.
  - Earliest sign in maceration is skin slippage (seen in 12 hours).
  - Blebs on skin contain red serous fluid.

- Body is soft, flaccid **and flattens out**.
- Most important sign of dead born child*.

Radiological Signs of Dead Born Child are:

- *Spalding's sign:* Loss of alignments overriding of bones of cranial vault, occurs due to shrinkage of the cerebrum. Little value before 20 weeks.
- *Robert's sign:*
  - ♦ Gas shadow in the heart chamber and blood vessels.
  - ♦ First radiological sign of infant death, seen in 12 hours.
- *Deuel's Halo sign:* Increase pericranial fat.
- *Ball sign/Blair Hartley sign: Hyperflexion* of spine.
- *Helix sign:* Gas in umbilical arteries.
- *Crowding* of ribs.

C. **Mummification** may be seen in the dead born fetus if there was:

- Deficient blood supply.
- Scanty liquor amnii.
- No air entry in uterus.

II. VIABILITY

- Physical ability of a fetus to lead "separate existence".
- A child is viable after 210 days (7×30 days).

Signs of Viability

1. Length → 35 cm (using Hasse's rule 7×5 = 35 cm).
2. Weight → 900 to 1200 gms.
3. Eyelids an open, pupillary membrane disappears.
4. Testies are found at external inguinal ring.
5. Ossification centres appearing at viability.
   - Centre for talus.
   - Centre for 2nd and 3rd piece of sternum.

III. LIVE BIRTH

Definition: A child showing signs of life even when only part of the child was out of the mother.

Signs of Live Birth

- Abdomen* is opened first before thorax during autopsy of an infant (in poisoning cases cranial cavity is opened first), to note level of diaphragm.

- The level of diaphragm is lower after respiration, at the level of 6th and 7th rib.

Vagitus Uterinus

The emotional turmoil which crying expresses can already exist in the womb and may be vocalized if air reaches the area around the fetal larynx. This intrauterine crying is termed "vagitus uterinus (literally, squalling in the womb) and is well documented in medical literature.

Test for Live Births

1. **Wreden's test:** For air in middle ear.
2. **Breslaus sign:** For air in stomach and duodenum.
3. **Fodere's test:** Weight of lungs:
   - 30 grams – still born.
   - 60 grams – live born.

   [Memorizer: Fodere's—Full weight]
4. **Ploquet's test:** Weight of lungs to body *(Wt of lungs increases due to blood flowing in them*).*

   1 : 70 unrespired lung.

   1 : 35 respired lung.

   [Memorizer: Ploquet's Proportional Ratio]
5. **Hydrostatic floatation test (Raygat's Test*/ Docimasy)**
   - Lungs float if the child has respired. Liver is used as control, if liver floats test is of no value.
   - Lungs are squeezed to remove tidal air.
   - Lung float due to residual air, as specific gravity of lungs decreases to **0.94**.

Fallacies

a. *Respired lungs may sink in certain conditions (False Negative)*
   - Pneumonia.
   - Acute edema.
   - *Alveolar duct membrane*.*

b. *Unrespired lungs may float in certain conditions (False Positive)*
   - Putrefaction.
   - Artificial respiration.

- Hydrostatic test is not necessary in case: **(Memorizer → 5 Ms)**
  1. Foetus is non-viable (<180 days)—Lack of **M**aturity.

2. Foetus is dead born (e.g., **M**aceration and **M**ummification).
3. Foetus is a **M**onster (Genetic deformity).
4. **M**ilk is present in stomach.
5. U**M**bilical cord is separated and scar is formed.

- Spongy and crepe tent lungs, is result of accumulation of gases in the lung thus hydrostatic test is not performed.

Other Signs of Live Birth are:

1. Caput secundum is present.
2. Cephal haematoma.
3. Umbilical artery obliterates in 3 days (Forms Medial umbilical fold).
4. Umbilical vein (left) obliterates in 4 days (Forms Ligamentum Teres).
5. Change in umbilical cord→falls off in 5-6 days. **[Remember→A3, V4, C5-6…3,4,5-6].**

- Most common site where the umbilical cord torn is the **fetal end***.

Important Sections

- Sec. 317 IPC **A**bandoning the fetus ***[A].***
- Sec. 318 IPC **C**oncealment of birth ***[B].***

Battered Baby Syndrome

- Also known as:
  - Caffey's syndrome (See also Cafe coronary).
  - Non-accidental injuries of childhood.
  - Inflicted Traumatic Brain Injury (ITBI).
  - Inflicted Childhood Neurotrauma (ICN).
- Features:
  - Inconsistent history and findings of physical examination **(Mismatch).**
  - Multiple bruises of different colours in same individual.**
  - Infantile whiplash syndrome: Acceleration and Deceleration Injuries (AC-DC).

The three most commonly found injuries in **Shaken Baby Syndrome** cases are:

1. Bleeding in and around the brain, also called **subdural** and sometimes subarachnoid hematomas.
2. Retinal hemorrhaging, or bleeding in the different layers of the back of the eye; during violent shaking episodes, the vitreous heaves and tears the blood vessels within the various layers of the retina. The resulting **"bleeds" are known as "dot" (smaller) or "blot" (larger)** hemorrhages. These are "**flame like**" in appearance [DOT and BLOT Hemorrhage].
3. Brain swelling, also known as cerebral edema.

Shaken baby syndrome is a leading cause of death in infants under the age of two years old.

X-rays: Multiple rib fractures, result in callus formation which give ***String of Beads*** appearance.

- **Posterior Rib Fractures :** Child's ribs break near the junction with the spine.
- **Classic Metaphyseal Lesions and Fractures**
  a. Bucket handle: Zone of growth is twisted.
  b. Corner fractures: Zone of growth moves sideways.
- **Egg Shell Fracture:** A skull fracture that radiates out in different directions.
- **Retraction Balls** due to diffuse axonal injuries may be seen in SBS.
- **Babygram** is used for diagnosis: A single X-ray of the entire body.

*Manchausan Syndrome of Proxy**

- Child is brought to hospital with repeated frivolous complaints by the parents.

SIDS

- Cot death or crib death.
- *Cause of death:* Most accepted hypothesis is "Sleep Apnoea".

MCQs

1. **Infanticide means unlawful destruction of a child under the age of:**
   A. 15 days **B.** One month
   C. 6 months **D.** One year
2. **Normally a foetus becomes viable by:**
   A. 170 days **B.** 180 days
   C. 200 days **D.** 210 days
3. **Spalding sign indicates:**
   A. Viable child **B.** Dead born child
   C. Still born child **D.** Live born child
4. **Hydrostatic test is not required in following cases:**
   A. Dead born **B.** Non-viable child
   C. Monster child **D.** All of the above
5. **After inspiration the weight of the lungs of a newly born child increase approximately by:**
   A. 10 grams **B.** 20 grams
   C. 30 grams **D.** 40 grams
6. **Aseptic autolysis is known as:**
   A. Maceration **B.** Decomposition
   C. Mummification **D.** Adipocere
7. **Stillborn child is above the gestation age of:**
   A. 20 weeks **B.** 24 weeks
   C. 28 weeks **D.** 36 weeks
8. **Live birth according to Indian law is when:**
   A. Any part of a living child comes out
   B. Child is completely out of mother's private parts
   C. Child is completely born and cries
   D. Child is completely born and shows signs of respiration

---

1 D 2 D 3 B 4 D 5 C 6 A 7 C 8 A

9. Specific gravity of lungs after start of respiration become:
A. 0.98
B. 0.94
C. 0.90
D. 0.84

10. Umbilical veins and ductus venosus obliterate after birth by:
A. 24 hours
B. 2nd day
C. 4th day
D. 10th day

11. Mummified umbilical cord fall off by:
A. 3rd day
B. 6th day
C. 10th day
D. 14th day

12. In a child, the level of foetal haemoglobin in the 3rd month goes down to:
A. 20%
B. 15%
C. 8%
D. 2%

13. The ossification center to confirm that foetus is viable is seen in:
A. Talus
B. Calcaneum
C. Lower end of femur
D. Upper end of tibia

14. Umbilical cord is torn in precipitate labour:
A. Near the foetal end
B. Near placental end
C. In the middle
D. Not torn

15. Caffey's syndrome pertains to:
A. Cot death
B. Sudden infant death syndrome
C. Choking deaths
D. Battered baby

9 B 10 C 11 B 12 C 13 A 14 A 15 D

16. Battered baby syndrome can be diagnosed by:

A. Injuries are of different age groups
B. Serious or grievous injuries are not seen
C. Prompt medical attention
D. Exclusively seen in male children

17. Most commonly accepted theory for the cause of SIDS is:

A. Respiratory infections
B. Allergic reaction to cow's milk
C. Sleep apnoea
D. Conduction defects in hearts

18. Injury commonly seen in a case of infantile whiplash syndrome is:

A. Subdural haematoma
B. Damage to cervical vertebrae
C. Laceration of liver
D. Bursting of urinary bladder

19. Length of 4 months old foetus is:

A. 12 cms **B.** 16 cms
C. 20 cms **D.** 25 cms

20. The hydrostatic test need not be performed in case of:

A. Infanticide
B. Spongy or crepitant
C. Lungs or liver like in consistency
D. None of the above

21. Spaldings sign is seen with..... foetus.

A. Live born
B. Dead born
C. Still born
D. All of the above

22. Macerated foetus indicates:

A. Dead born **B.** Still born
C. Live born **D.** IUGR

16 A 17 C 18 A 19 B 20 B 21 B 22 A

23. Spaldings sign is diagnostic of:

A. Prematurity B. Post maturity
C. Fetal death D. Hydrocephalus

24. Mummification is seen in dead born fetus:

A. Scanty liquor amnii
B. Deficient blood supply
C. No air entry to uterus
D. All of the above

25. Postmortem in a newborn baby is done by opening first:

A. The skull
B. The chest cavity
C. The abdominal cavity
D. Any of the above according to convenience

26. The currently favoured hypothesis suggests that cot-deaths are due to:

A. Allergy to cow's milk protein
B. Laryngeal spasm
C. Prolonged sleep apnoea
D. Respiratory infection

27. Ductus arteriosus completely obliterates in:

A. 24-72 hours
B. 3-6 days
C. 6-12 days
D. 2-4 weeks

28. Legal age by which fetus is capable of independent existence is:

A. 240 days B. 230 days
C. 220 days D. 210 days

29. Aseptic autolysis is seen in:

A. Maceration
B. Mummification
C. Adipocere
D. Putrefaction

---

23 C 24 D 25 C 26 C 27 A 28 D 29 A

30. In prenatal diagnostic technique Act 1994 which one of the following is not a ground for carrying out prenatal test?

A. Pregnant women above 35 years

B. History of two or more spontaneous abortion or fetal loss

C. When fetal heart rate is 160 per min at fifth and 120 per min at ninth

D. History of exposure to potentially teratogenic drugs

31. A dead born foetus does not have:

A. Rigor mortis at birth

B. Adipocere formation

C. Maceration

D. Mummification

30 C 31 B

7 Thermal Injuries

Injuries Due to Very Low Temperature

Generalised Effect: Hypothermia

- When temperature falls below 35°C it is called hypothermia.
- Below 30°C hypothalamus fails to regulate temperature.
- **Fat Necrosis of Pancreas** is the most characteristic findings of thermal injuries.

Local Effects

- **Trench foot** and **Immersion foot** are the result of prolonged exposure to severe cold (5 to 8°C) and dampness.*

Frost Bite—Exposure to extreme cold (-2.5°C temperature. In frostbite, **skin** becomes hard and black in 2 weeks.

Erythema Pernio (Chilblain)

Red, itchy skin lesions associated with edema and blistering due to exposure to cold.

Paradoxical Undressing

- Occurs in moderate to severe **Hypothermia.**
- Person becomes disoriented, starts discarding his clothes which increase the temperature loss.
- This phenomenon can be confused with death (homicide) after sexual assault.

Hide and Die Phenomenon

- Seen in Hypothermia.
- Person under mental confusion and hibernation reflex tries to hide oneself in strange places.
- This phenomenon can be confused with death (homicide) after burglary and robbery.

HEAT

Generalised Effects

1. **Heat cramps** (miner's cramps or fireman's cramps). They are caused by rapid **dehydration** of body through the loss of water and salt in the sweat. Muscle cramp is due to loss of Na^+ ion.
2. **Heat hyperpyrexia or Heat stroke**
   - The term **'Thermic fever or Sunstroke'** is used when there has been direct exposure to the sun.
   - High temperature, increased humidity, minor infections, muscular activity and lack of acclimatization are the principal factors in initiation.
   - Failure of cutaneous blood flow and sweating leads to breakdown of heat regulating center of hypothalamus.
   - Breathing is rapid, deep and **Kussmaul** type.
   - Edema and reduction of Purkinje's cells in cerebellum is the **most important finding** in autopsy.
3. **Heat prostration** (heat exhaustion and heat syncope)
   - Heat prostration is a condition of collapse **without increase in body temperature**, which follows exposure to excessive heat.
   - Main cause of death is **vascular collapse and syncope.**

Local Effects

Burns

- A burn is an injury, which is caused by application of heat or chemical substances to the external or internal surfaces of the body.
- **Necklacing** is a method of homicidal burning developed in **South African** townships; it involves placing a vehicle tyre around the neck of the victim.
- Vacuolisation in epidermal and dermal layers is a characteristic feature of burns.
- **Degrees of Burns**
  - **Dupuytren** recognized *six degrees** of burns but they were merged into three groups by **Wilson.**

1. **Epidermal** (First and second degree Dupuytren)
   - Usually a blister (vesicle or bulla) is formed which is covered by white, avascular epidermis, bordered by red, hyperaemic skin.
   - These burns are very painful.
   - Repair is complete without scar formation*.
2. **Dermo-epidermal** (3rd and 4th degree Dupuytren)
   - Whole thickness of skin is destroyed.
   - Skin and subcutaneous tissue is affected.
   - In dermo-epidermal, pain and shock are greater than in first degree burns (*most painful*).**
3. **Deep** (5th and 6th degree Dupuytren)
   - In this, there is gross destruction not only of the skin and subcutaneous tissue but also of muscles and even bone.
   - Nerve endings are also destroyed and as such, the burns are relatively painless.***
   - **The extent of the surface**
     - The estimation of the surface area of the body involved is worked out by the **'rule of nine'** by Wallace*.
     - **Rule of Palm:** In case of patchy burns, rule of '9' is of less value. Palm of an individual is 1% of the Body Surface Area.
     - Minimum **1/3rd** area must be involved to label it grievous*.
     - Genitals constitute 0% of surface area up to 9 years.
     - Head forms the largest area in children.

- Minimum **1/3rd** area must be involved to label it grievous*.

To memorize–Rule of "five" [Approximation of Lund and Browder Chart]	
Infants	*Older children*
Head + Neck+ Face = 20% Trunk 40% (front 20% + back 20%) Each Limb 10%	Head + Neck + Face 15% Front of trunk 20% Back of trunk 15% Each lower limb 15% Each upper limb 10%

Parkland formula is used to calculate the fluid to be given in the first 24 hours.

- **Causes of death**
  - i. Primary (neurogenic) shock due to pain.
  - ii. More than half of deaths from burns occur from secondary shock due to fluid loss from burnt surface.
  - iii. Toxaemia.
  - iv. Sepsis.
  - v. Acute renal failure pyemia.
  - vi. Suffocation.

- **Difference between Antemortem and Postmortem Burns**

Trait	*Antemortem*	*Postmortem burns*
1. Line of redness	i. Present	i. Absent
2. Blister	ii. Contains serous fluid with proteins and chlorides. Base is inflamed	ii. Contains air only. Base is dry hard and yellow
3. Vital reaction	iii. Present	iii. Absent
4. Enzymes	iv. Increase in enzyme reaction and SH group	iv. Does not show increase in enzyme reaction
5. CO Hb	v. More than 5% of CO Hb	v. Less

- Teeth become loose in their socket in antemortem burns.
- **Puppet Organs:** Heat causes fixation and shrinkage of the internal organs which become firm, shrunken so-called 'puppet organs'.

- Red blood cell fragmentation and haemolysis causes **an intense red discoloration of the intima of blood vessels** similar to that which occurs during normal putrefaction.
- **Presence of** soot particles in trachea and an **elevated CO saturation** together are absolute proof that the victim was **Alive** when fire occurred.
- Cyanide levels are elevated in thermal death.
- **Heat haematoma**
  - It resembles *extra-dural haemorrhage**.
  - Clot has **honey comb*** appearance, light chocolate colour.
  - Most common site parietotemporal region.

Heat Rupture can be Confused with Incised Wounds

Heat rupture [H.R.] is characterized by:

a. Absence of blood clots.
b. Blood vessels are not burst but stretched across fissures (intact vessels with coagulated blood).
c. Edges are irregular.
d. Presence of tissue bridges.
e. HR are more commonly seen at the extensor surfaces and joints.

- **Thermal Fracture**
  - They do not cross suture lines.
- **Street-and-Avenue Fractures:** Thermal fractures of long bones may appear arc-shaped on the surface or occasionally as 'street-and-avenue fractures' composed of jagged lines of fracture at right angles to each other.
- **Pugilistic attitude** (boxing, fencing or defence attitude).
- Pugilistic attitude is due to heat stiffening, **seen both in AM and PM burns***.
  - Coagulation of protein albumin of the muscles which causes contraction and thus responsible for pugilistic attitude.
- Heat stiffening is due to exposure of the body to temperature above **75°C.**
- Pugilistic attitude is seen in those dying due to burns and sudden immersion in boiling liquid.

- In heat stiffening, body assumes a posture of generalized flexion. Elbows, hip and knee joints flexed. Fingers clawed like hooks (Forensic Imager).
- **Curling Ulcers** are seen in duodenum.

Inhalation Injuries

Mechanisms by which smoke inhalation produces respiratory damage leading to **Hypoxaemia** are:

- Thermal injury to the respiratory tract.
- Carbon monoxide poisoning.
- Direct particulate injury.
- Smoke poisoning.

Carboxy Hb is estimated by spectroscopic methods making use of the fact that oxyhaemoglobin and COHb have different absorption spectra.

The result is expressed as the percentage saturation and is the ratio of COHb to total haemoglobin × 100.

The effects of COHb at different percentage saturation

0-10%	:	No immediate ill effects
10-20%	:	Dizziness and shortness of breath on exertion
20-30%	:	Dizziness, headache, nausea and fatigue
30-40%	:	Impaired judgement, unconsciousness may occur
40-60%	:	**Unconsciousness and death likely**

- **Kunkel's Test for Carbon Monoxides.**

Cyanide Effect in Fire

- Normal blood cyanide levels are less than 8 μmol/L.
- Non-fatal toxic effects begin at about 50 μmol/L.
- Fatal threshold is above 100 μmol/L.

[**cf.** A suicide technique that mixes household chemicals to produce a deadly **Hydrogen Sulphide** gas became a grisly fad in Japan, became popular over internet as **Dangerous Japanese 'Detergent Suicide' Technique]**.

Scalds

- A scald is an injury, which is caused by application of liquid above **60°C** or from stream.

(Remember **"6 Tea"** cups are thrown on someone cause scalds, Hot !!).

- Skin becomes sodden and bleached.
- Clothes are wet but not burnt.

Chemical Burns

VITRIOLAGE (Vitriol throwing): Throwing of acid on another individual is known as vitriolage. It leads to chemical burns. It comes under Sec. 320 IPC (Grievous hurt/Sixth clause).

i. Acid Burns:

- Acids with a pH less than 2 precipitate proteins causing coagulation necrosis.
- Acid burns are clearly demarcated, dry and with a leathery scab.

> **The colour of scab**
> - Nitric acid: Yellow-brown scab.
> - Sulphuric (vitriol): Black-brown scab.
> - Hydrochloric acid (spirit of salt): **White to Grey scab***.
> - Carbolic acid (phenol or lysol): Light brown scab.

ii. Alkali Burns: [Memorizer→AlkaLI (LIquefactive)]

- Alkalis with a pH above 11.5 cause more tissue damage than acids because they induce **Liquefactive Necrosis**, which facilitates ever deeper penetration of the alkali.
- The caustic alkalis, such as sodium hydroxide (caustic soda or lye) and ammonium hydroxide, leave a **Grey-White mucoid burn.**

Chemical Warfare

Some chemical warfare agents produce skin burns.

i. Mustard Gas

- Best known vesicants.
- Also known as sulphur **mustard**, named because its garlic or mustard smell.

- First used during World War I.
- It is an incapacitating agent with a mortality rate of 2-3%.
- Deaths are the result of respiratory effects or bone marrow depression with associated infections.
- **Blisters** are characteristic of mustard gas, by contrast with acids and alkalis which do not produce blistering when they burn the skin. These blisters are uncomfortable but not painful, although they are delicate and easily rubbed off, leaving the now painful blister base.
- When exposure is severe, the first sign is **Striking Erythema**, reminiscent of scarlet fever. As the erythema fades, areas of hyperpigmentation are left behind, as occurs with sunburn.

ii. **Lewisite** is another chemical warfare agent which, like mustard, is a vesicant. It is non-persistent, so attacks can be launched on previously contaminated ground. Lewisite is ineffective under wet conditions.

iii. **Phenyldichlorarsine** was used on a large scale during World War I because it was capable of penetrating the respirators available that time.

High Explosives are of Two Categories

(i) **Initiating explosives**

Very sensitive and have the potential for unexpected detonation home-manufactured bombs rarely use initiating explosives.

E.g.: Mercury Fulminate, Lead Azide.

(ii) **Non-initiating explosives** Less sensitive and more commonly used in commercial and military applications.

E.g.

- **Dynamite** (based on Nitroglycerine).
- **TNT** (trinitrotoluene).
- **RDX** (Penta Erythritrol Tetra-Nitrate) also known as Research and Development Explosive.

- **PETN** (cyclotrimethylenetrinitramine).
- **ANFO,** Ammonium Nitrate and Fuel Oil. Ammonium nitrate is an oxygen-rich oxidant that can be found in fertilizers, commonly used in terrorist attacks.

Electrical Injuries

Electrocution:

- The mechanism of death is most commonly a cardiac dysrhythmia, usually ventricular fibrillation, sometimes paralysis of the respiratory muscles, and rarely a direct effect on the brainstem.
- It can lead to suspended animation.
- Skin burns is a pathognomonic marker for death by electrocution.

Type of Electrical Burns

a. **Joule Burn (contact electrical burns).**
b. Spark (arc) type.

a. Joule Burn (Endogenous Burns)

1. Firm contact electrical burns.
2. Entry typically leaves a **central collapsed blister**, which may reproduce the shape of the conductor, with a surrounding areola of pallor. The blister is created by steam, and when the current ceases, **the blister cools and collapses to leave a crater** with a raised rim.
3. With the passage of an electric current, metallic ions from the metal conductor combine with tissue anions to form **Metallic salts** which are deposited, and may be demonstrated by **chemical, histochemical and spectrographic techniques.**
4. **Histology:** Cellular Eosinophilia and Nuclear Streaming.
5. In high-voltage (more than 1,000 volts) electrical burns the contact injury of exit often appears as a blow-out type of wound.

b. Spark (Arc) Burn:

1. Occurs when there is an **air gap** between the conductor and the skin so that the current arcs across the gap as a spark.

2. The extremely high temperature of sparks causes the epidermal keratin to melt and, after cooling, this leaves a raised brown or yellow nodule of fused keratin surrounded by an areola of pale skin.
3. **High voltage spark burns** may cause large areas of skin damage resulting in an appearance of **'Crocodile Skin'.**
4. The severity of the electrical injury to the deep tissues depends upon the **Amperage**, i.e., the actual amount of current passing through the tissues.
5. **Electrical Resistance of Tissues:** Bone (166 Omega Metres) > Fat > Dry skin > Wet skin

Quick Recap
• **Joule Burn** is specific and diagnostic of contact electrical burn. • Joule burn is **endogenous burn.** • **Crocodile flash burns** are due to high voltage burns. These are multiple disc rate lesions due to **'Arc Effect'.** • **Acro-Reaction Test:** A micro chemical test for metals at the site of entry of electric current leading to deposition of metal particles in the skin. • Death occurs from ventricular fibrillation. • **Current Pearls and wax drippings** are important autopsy finding. • Skeletal fractures and joint dislocations may occur as a result of **Tetanic Contractions.** • Skeletal muscle damage leads to release of myoglobin, and muscle-specific intracellular enzymes, with resultant **Myoglobinaemia and Myoglobinuria in survivors.** • An unusual and characteristic finding in **electrocution in the bath** is that the subsequent development of **hypostasis (postmortem lividity)** is limited by the **WATER-LINE**, resulting in a stark and unusual demarcation. • Judicial execution by electricity was first done in New York in 1890.

Lightning Stroke

- A flash of lightning is due to an electrical discharge from a cloud to the earth.
- Arborescent burns are superficial, irregular, thin, resembling the branches of a tree*, also called **Litchenberg's** flowers, Keraunographic Markings or **Filligree burns.**
- Most common site is shoulder flanks. They tend to follow skin creases and the long axis of the body.
- *These figures disappear after 24 hours, if victim survives.*
- *Cause of* ***filligree burns:*** Staining of tissues with hemoglobin, along the path of current.

> **PQZ→Mechanism:** Lightening Injuries inflicted by **high voltage lightning** or electric shock. **Litchenberg's** flowers are skin lesions in the form of tree-like reddish-brown patterns arranged on the surface of the skin. It is due to:
> **(a) Paralysis of Capillaries.**
> **(b) Thermal Denaturation of Erythrocytes***.

Sledge Hammer Effect: Lightning Injuries

According to Spencer there are 4 factors that result in injury in a lightning flash:

- Direct effect of high voltage current.
- Burning by super heated air.
- Effect of expanded and repelled air; and
- **Sledge Hammer Effect:**
  - Blow dealt by compressed air pushed before the current produced by lightning.
  - Bruising is usually at the back of head.

MCQs

1. Pugilistic attitude in burns is seen in:
- **A.** Antemortem burns
- **B.** Postmorten burns
- **C.** Homicidal burns
- **D.** Suicidal burns
- **E.** Both antemortem burns and postmortem burns

2. Joule burn is seen in:
- **A.** Electrocution
- **B.** Thermal injury
- **C.** Radiation injury
- **D.** Lightning

3. Puglistic attitude is seen in:
- **A.** Drowning
- **B.** Protein coagulation
- **C.** Electrocoagulation
- **D.** Hanging

4. Pugilistic attitude is due to:
- **A.** Burns
- **B.** Vitriolage
- **C.** Flexor group contracture
- **D.** Extensor group contracture

5. More than 5% carboxyhaemoglobin is indicative of:
- **A.** Antemortem burns
- **B.** Drowning
- **C.** HCN poisoning
- **D.** Suffocation

6. In a completely charred body at autopsy, medical officer can say that the burns are antemortem if he can find:
- **A.** Soot in respiratory passage
- **B.** Cyanosis of finger nails
- **C.** Congestion of kidney
- **D.** Pale internal organs

1 E 2 A 3 B 4 A 5 A 6 A

7. Following are the causes of death in a patient with burns *except:*
A. Shock **B.** Suffocation
C. Sepsis **D.** Air embolism

8. For hydrostatic test to be positive at all stages, the following must be present inside lung alveoli:
A. Residual air
B. Tidal air
C. Exudates and tidal air
D. Amniotic fluid and tidal air

9. Filigree burns are due to:
A. Chemicals
B. Lightning
C. Electric shock
D. Radiation burns

10. In frost bite, skin becomes hard and black in about:
A. 3 days **B.** 7 days
C. 2 weeks **D.** 4-6 weeks

11. Gas in great vessels of foetus indicate:
A. Fetal distress
B. Post mature fetus
C. Fetal death
D. Premature fetus

12. Crocodile skin appearance is seen in:
A. High voltage burns **B.** Electric shock
C. Drowning **D.** Mummifications

13. Filigree burns are due to:
A. Splashes **B.** Flame burns
C. AC current **D.** Lightning

14. Elevated levels of cyanide is seen in death due to which of the following?
A. Cold **B.** Scald
C. Starvation **D.** Thermal burns

7 D 8 A 9 B 10 C 11 C 12 A 13 D 14 D

8

Forensic Psychiatry

Paolo Zachhia is regarded as the father of Forensic Psychiatrist.

Delirium

- Delusions and Hallucinations are present.
- It occurs in physical disease with high fever, overwork, mental stress, metabolic disease, cerebral neoplasm or drug intoxication.
- Such persons are not responsible for their criminal acts.

Delusion (Disorder of Cognition/Belief)

- Delusion is a false belief in something, which is not a fact, and which persists even after its falsity has been clearly demonstrated.
- It is a disorder of thought/cognition.
- *Types:*
  i. *Grandeur or exaltation:* A man imagines himself to be very rich while in reality he is a pauper.
  ii. *Persecution:* Person believes that people, things events etc. refer to him in a special way.
  iii. *Influence:* His thought, feelings and actions are being influenced and controlled by some outside agencies.
  iv. *Infidelity:* A man imagines his wife to be unfaithful while in fact she is chaste.

v. *Nihilistic:* The person declares that he does not exist or that there is no world seen in major depression.
vi. *Hypochondriac:* The person believes that there is something wrong with his body, though in fact he is healthy.
vii. *Capgras Syndrome:* Person believes that someone close to oneself has been replaced by exact double.
viii. *Fregoli's Phenomenon:* Strangers are identified as familiar people.
ix. *Cotard Syndrome:* Person has delusion that he is dead, does not exist, putrefying etc.

Hallucination

- Hallucination is a **false sense of perception** without any external object or stimulus to produce it. They are purely imaginary and may effect any or all the special sense organs.
- **Types:**
  1. *Visual:* A person imagines of being attacked by a lion when no lion exists.
  2. *Auditory:* A person hears voices, when no one is present.
  3. *Olfactory:* A person smells pleasant or unpleasant odour when none is present.
  4. ***Tactile*****:* A man imagines rats and mice crawling into his bed, e.g., Magnan's symptoms.
- Hallucinations occur in fevers, intoxications and insanity.
- Visual and auditory hallucinations are most common.
- A person suffering from unpleasant hallucination may commit suicide or homicide.
- Olfactory hallucination is seen in temporal epilepsy.

Illusion

- Illusion is **false interpretation** by the senses of an external object or stimulus which has a real existence, e.g., A lion for a dog, or hears the notes of birds to human voice, imagines a string to be snake, stem of a tree for a ghost in dark.

- A sane person may experience illusion, but is capable of correcting the false impressions.
- An insane person continues to believe in the illusions even though the real facts are clearly pointed out.

E.g. of illusion

1. 2.

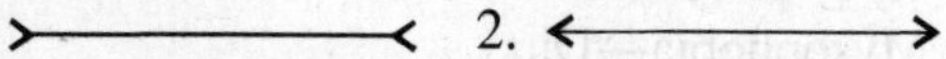

Line 1 appears longer than line 2 due to visual illusion.

Impulse

- This is a sudden and irresistible force compelling a person to the conscious performance of some action without motive or forethought.
- A sane person is capable of controlling an impulse, but an insane person may do things on impulse.
- **Types:**
  1. **Kleptomania**–An irresistible desire to steal articles of little value.
  2. **Pyromania**–An irresistible desire to set fire to things.
  3. **Multilomania**–An irresistible desire to mutilate animals.
  4. **Dipsomania**–An irresistible desire for alcoholic drinks at periodic intervals.
  5. **Oniomania:** Compulsive desire for shopping.
  6. **Irresistible impulse test (New Hempshire Test):**

     Criminal responsibility and impulse disorder.

Obsession

- In this a single idea, thought or emotion is constantly entertained by a person, which he recognizes as irrational, but persists in spite of all efforts to drive it from his mind.

- It is a disorder of **content of thought.**

Phobia

- It is an excessive or irrational fear of a particular object or situation.
  Agoraphobia→Opcn spaces
  Claustrophobia→Closed spaces
  Acrophobia→High spaces
  Nyctophobia→Darkness
  Mysophobia→Dirt.

Lucid Interval

- This is a period occurring in insanity during which all the symptoms of insanity disappear completely.
- The individual is able to judge his acts soundly and he becomes legally liable for his acts.
- If he commits an offence, he cannot be completely held responsible because it is difficult to know whether he was suffering from some mental abnormality at the time of committing the offence.
- **Oneiroid state** is state of mental confusion, amnesia, illusion and anxiety.
- It occurs in Delirium and early Schizophrenia.

Psychopath

- A person who is neither insane nor mentally defective, but fails to conform to normal standards of behaviour.

Mental Subnormality

1. Idiocy—I.Q. is 0-20.
2. Imbecility—I.Q. is 20-50.
3. Feeble minded—I.Q. is 20-50.
4. Normal I.Q.
   - It is more than 90.
   - Mental retardation is I.Q. less than 70.
   - I.Q. = (M.A./C.A.) × 100.
     (M.A.=Mental age; C.A.=Chronological age)

Difference between Real Insanity and Feigned Insanity

Trait	*Real Insanity*	*Feigned Insanity*
1. Onset	Gradual	Sudden
2. Motive	Absent	Present
3. Predisposing factors	Usually present e.g. H/o of insanity in parents or sudden monetary loss, grief etc.	Absent
4. Signs and symptoms	Uniform and present whether the patient is being observed or not	Presently only when conscious of being observed
5. Facial expres-sions	Peculiar e.g. Vacant look or fixed look of excitement	No peculiarity
6. Onsomnia	Present	Cannot persist
7. Exertion	Patient can stand exertion of fatigue, hunger, sleep	Breaks down with exertion
8. Habits	Dirty and filthy	Not dirty and filthy
9. Skin and lips	Dry, harsh	Normal
10. Frequent	Does not mind examination	Resents from fear of detection

- **The Mental Health Act, 1987**
  - Indian Lunacy Act was passed in 1912. It was repealed by the Mental Health Act, 1987.
- **Diagnosis of Insanity**
  - Individual should be kept for observation till 10 days.
  - Only with the permission of Magistrate a person can be detained upto 30 days.
  - Certificate can be issued after **minimum 3 examinations by two doctors**.

Mental Disorder and Responsibility

- Responsibility, in the legal sense means the liability of a person for his acts or omissions, and if these are against the law, the liability to be punished for them.

Civil Responsibility

- Insanity and Testamentary capacity–**Testamentary capacity** (Testament = will) is the mental ability of a person to make a valid will.
- **Holographic Will:** A will written by the testator in his/her own handwriting.
- The requirement of a valid will as follows:
  - A written and properly signed and witnessed document must exist.
- A person with **sound disposing mind*** (at the time of making will/NOT always) can make a valid will.

Evidence: Insane person can give evidence during lucid interval.

Criminal Responsibility

- The law presumes that for every criminal act, there must be criminal intent or mind = **mens rea** (mens = mind; rea = criminal) motivating it.
- The following are the tests for **judging criminal responsibility.**
  1. Mc Naughten rule (the Right or wrong test*; the Legal test)
     a. English courts, in dealing with the responsibility of the insane in criminal cases are guided by the rules laid down after the Mc Naughten trail in 1843.
     b. The most important aspect of this rule is as follows:
        - An accused person is not criminally responsible, if it is proved at the time of committing the crime that he was suffering from such a defect of reason from disease of mind that he did not know the nature and quality of act he is doing.
        - This legal test has also been accepted in India as the **law of criminal responsibilities under Sec 84 IPC.**

Defect: In McNaughten's Rule only intellectual factors are considered but emotions, delusion and control of impulses is ignored.

2. Durham Rule (1954).
3. Curren's Rule (1964).
4. The Irresistible Impulse Test.
5. The American Law Institute Test (1970).
6. Brawner Rule (1972).

Drunkenness

1. **Section 85 IPC** deals with the criminal responsibility of intoxicated person.
2. An intoxicated person (voluntary drunkenness) is criminally responsible if he has intention or knowledge of committing a crime (Sec 86 IPC).
3. A person is not criminally responsible during:
   - Post traumatic automalism.
   - Twilight.
   - Oneroid state.

Parasuicide

- Also known as Attempted Suicide or Pseudicide.
- Term coined by Norman Kreitman.
- The most common method–Overdose of Medicines/drugs.

Sec 328 and Sec. 329 Cr. PC deals with the procedure of examination of a mentally ill person.

MCQs

1. **Mental Health Act 1987 deals with such individuals, which are known as:**
   A. Lunatics B. Mad
   C. Mentally ill D. Insane
2. **A delusion is the disorder of:**
   A. Thought
   B. Orientation
   C. Perception
   D. Reasoning
3. **Hallucination is:**
   A. False interpretation of a stimulus
   B. False belief
   C. False sense perception without a stimulus
   D. Irresistible desire
4. **Obsession is appearance of persistent and irresistible:**
   A. Thought B. Emotion
   C. Impulse D. All of the above
5. **Pyromania is a type of:**
   A. Obsession B. Impulse
   C. Delusion D. Phobia
6. **According to Indian legal system I.Q. of an imbecile is between:**
   A. 0-20 B. 20-50
   C. 50-70 D. 80-100
7. **For diagnosis of mental illness a person can be kept under medical observation maximum upto:**
   A. 7 days B. 15 days
   C. 30 days D. 60 days

---

1 C 2 A 3 C 4 D 5 B 6 B 7 C

8. A mentally ill person who has escaped from psychiatric hospital can be retaken if caught within:

A. 10 days B. 20 days
C. 30 days D. 60 days

9. In schizophrenia, which of the following is disturbed?

A. Affect (feeling)
B. Cognition (Thinking)
C. Perception
D. All of the above

10. Schizophrenia like psychosis may be seen with chronic use of:

A. Alcohol B. Amphetamines
C. Charas D. Brown sugar

11. If at the time of marriage, either of them was incapable of giving valid consent because of mental illness. The other party can get:

A. The marriage declared null and void
B. A divorce
C. Cannot get a divorce
D. A separation order

12. Testamentary capacity of an individual refers to:

A. Capacity to give evidence in a court
B. Capacity to file a case in the court
C. Make a valid will
D. Capacity to attest a document

13. To make a will legally valid:

A. It must always be attested by any two witnesses
B. A doctor should always be one of the witness
C. Individual should always be compos mentis
D. Individual should be of sound disposing mind at the time of making will

---

8 C 9 D 10 B 11 A 12 C 13 D

14. Section of IPC dealing with criminal responsibility of mentally ill person is:

A. 84 IPC B. 304 IPC
C. 44 IPC D. 320 IPC

15. McNaughten's rule is also known as:

A. Irresistible impulse rule
B. Right or wrong test
C. Inability to adhere to the right
D. Loss of capacity to obey the law

16. A person is held responsible for his acts done under following condition:

A. Delirium tremens
B. Epileptic condition
C. Hypnosis
D. Somnambulism

17. Lucid interval is seen in:

A. Insanity
B. Malignant disease
C. Electrical shock
D. Pyphilis

18. McNaughten's rule is concerned with:

A. Criminal responsibility
B. Litigation
C. Rape
D. Suicide

19. Which of the following legislation is regarding insanity?

A. McNaughten rule
B. Curren rule
C. Durnams rule
D. All of the above

20. Criminal responsibility of a person of unsound mind in India is incorporated in the Indian Penal Code:

A. Section 302 B. Section 84
C. Section 85 D. Section 88

---

14 A 15 B 16 C 17 A 18 A 19 D 20 B

21. Indian Lunacy Act was passed in:
A. 1804 B. 1912
C. 1916 D. 1921

22. Mental retardation is defined when I.Q. is below:
A. 90 B. 80
C. 70 D. 65

23. For diagnosis of lunacy a person can be kept under observation at a stretch for:
A. 2 days B. 7 days
C. 10 days D. 30 days

24. Mc Naughten's rule:
A. Section 84
B. Section 85
C. Section 86
D. Section 87

21 B 22 C 23 C 24 A

9

Starvation

- In **acute starvation**, there is a feeling of hunger for the first 30 to 48 hours, followed by pain in the epigastrium.
- After 4 to 5 days of starvation, general emaciation and absorption of the subcutaneous fat begins to occur.
- Before death body has offensive odour.
- Usually the loss of 40% of body weight is fatal.
- Death occurs from exhaustion, circulatory failure due to brown atrophy of the heart, or inter current infection.
- During starvation the substance which heart uses as energy source is aceto acetate.
- If starvation exceeds 7 days then the major nutrition supply of brain comes from ketone bodies.
- The changes in starvation seen are Hypoglycemia, Hypothermia, Hyper triglyceremia and Keto-acidosis.
- **On P-M examination**, the heart is small from brown atrophy, and chambers are empty.
- Brain is the **only organ** which do not show reduction in size and weight.
- Stress fractures are present.
- **Gallbladder is distended** with bile.

MCQs

1. **In starvation, the gallbladder may be:**
   A. Atrophied
   B. Distended
   C. Show stones
   D. Normal

2. **In an acute starvation feeling of intense hunger lasts:**
   A. 12-24 hours
   B. 24-36 hours
   C. 36-48 hours
   D. 48-60 hours

3. **Entire absence of fat throughout the body is suggestive of:**
   A. Starvation
   B. Tuberculosis
   C. Diabetes
   D. All of the above

4. **In acute starvation, feeling of intense hunger lasts:**
   A. 10 to 20 hours
   B. 20 to 30 hours
   C. 36 to 48 hours
   D. Beyond 60 hours

5. **If both water and food are completely withheld to a person, death usually occurs in:**
   A. 1 to 2 days
   B. 2 to 4 days
   C. 5 to 7 days
   D. 10 to 12 days

1 B 2 C 3 A 4 C 5 D

10
Biological Evidence

A. BLOOD

Medicolegal Questions in Relation to Blood Stains

1. **Blood effused in life** will form scales on drying, while after death blood tends to break up into powder.
2. **Blood or not**

   Presumptive Chemical Tests: These are based on an **oxidation-reduction reaction** in which a reagent (o-tolidine, tetramethylbenzidine, phenolphthalein and leucomalachite green) is oxidized by **hydrogen peroxide** (H_2O_2) in the presence of **Peroxidases** (which **Blood** has).

   i. **Benzidine Test/Rudolf Adler Test** *(No longer used as Benzidine is **Carcinogenic**):*
   - Most reliable chemical test for blood.
   - Add a drip of saturated solution of benzidine glacial acetic acid and then a drop of 10 volumes hydrogen peroxide.
   - If blood is present, dark blue colour is produced immediately.
   - A positive reaction is given by blood of almost any age, blood that has been exposed to heat or cold. It detects blood when present in a dilution of one part of blood in 3 lakhs and can detect blood which 100-150 years old.

- If a negative reaction is obtained it is certain that the stain is not blood.

(**Modern Variant–Combur Test:** The strips are impregnated with organic hydroperoxide and **tetramethylbenzidine** as a colourmetric indicator; if haemoglobin is present, causing oxidation, the strips turn from yellow to green-blue.)

ii. **Kastle Meyer's Test:**
- Also known as Phenolphthalein test.
- Extremely delicate.
- Pink colour if blood is present.

iii. **O-Toulidine Test:** Blood gives blue colour reaction.

iv. **Leuco Malachite Test:** Peacock-Blue colour.

v. **Guaiacum Test:** Deep blue.

vi. **Luminol Spray Test:** In this test, luminol powder ($C_8H_7O_3N_3$) **APH**: ***o*-Amino-phthaloyl-hydrazide** is mixed with hydrogen peroxide (H_2O_2) and Potassium hydroxide in a spray bottle. The iron from the hemoglobin in the blood serves as a catalyst for the chemiluminescence reaction that causes luminol to glow Blue. Useful to demonstrate faint/old washed up blood stains.

3. **Human Blood or Not**
- **An immunological method involving antigens and antibodies was discovered by Paul Uhlenhuth** (Precipitin Test).
- Precipitin test +ive in dead body up to 10 years.
- Precipitin test–This determines whether the blood is derived from human beings or from a lower animal.

4. **Micro Chemical Examination**

a. **Red corpuscles–Human RBCs are Biconcave, circular, non-nucleated.**

b. **Haemin crystal test (Teichamnn's Test)**– A small crystal of sodium chloride* and to 3 drops glacial acetic acid* are placed on a glass slide. Brownish-black rhombic crystals of haemin or haematin chloride arranged singly or in clusters are seen if blood is present. Teichman's Test is negative if stain is old, while Takayama is positive.

c. **Haemochromogen crystal test (Takayama test):** It has MORE value.
Stain + 2-3 drops of Takayama reagent (Sodium hydroxide + Pyridine + Glucose).
Pink feathery crystals of Haemochromogen.
[**Confusion Killer*** :::: only one **CH** in a row/column]

Takayama's test (No CH)	Haemo**CH**romogen (have CH)
TieCHamann's test (have CH)	Haemin crystal test (No CH)

d. ***Magrath test*:** If blood is present, luminescence is seen.

e. **Absorption spectroscopy *the most reliable, specific and most delicate test.***

General Concept: Confirmatory tests are **less sensitive** than presumptive and species-origin tests. Therefore, it is possible to obtain a negative result for a confirmatory test in the presence of blood. Hence, a **negative confirmatory test does not negate the presence of blood.**

5. **Blood Groups**

- **Karl Landsteiner** discovered the ABO blood group.
- **ABO group** can be demonstrated in all body fluids except **CSF.**
- **Bernstein's one gene-three allelic model** explains Inheritance of Blood Groups.
- **The Bombay Blood Group** is termed as 'OH', which means absence of 'H'.
- **Recent Blood Stain:** Direct Agglutination Test.
- **Old Blood Stain:** Absorption Elution Test.

Determining Possible Genotypes from Phenotypes

Phenotype	Possible Genotypes
A	AA or AO
B	BB or BO
AB	AB
O	OO

6. **Bloodstains are classified into three basic types:**
   1. Passive stains.
   2. Transfer stains; and
   3. Projected or Impact stains.

   Plasma vs. Serum
   Plasma is the liquid portion of whole, unclotted blood that contains proteins involved in the clotting process.
   Serum is the liquid that remains after the blood's proteins have clotted the blood.

B. SALIVA

Saliva is rich in the enzyme alpha-amylase (also known as α-amylase, salivary amylase, or Ptyalin. Mueller conceived the use of alpha-amylase as a forensic target to validate the presence of saliva on a given surface.

a. **Phadebas Test** is a presumptive test for alpha-amylase.
   Limitation: This test alone cannot confirm the presence of human saliva because this presumptive test will give a positive result if the alpha-amylase enzyme from *any organism* is present.
b. **Lateral Flow Immunochromatographic Strip Test** or Rapid Stain Identification (RSID) Saliva kits, use monoclonal antibodies to test molecule of Alpha-Amylase.

DNA Forensics

- Dr. Alec Jeffreys, used Restriction Fragment Length Polymorphism (RFLP) to analyze DNA.

- Variable Number of Tandem Repeats (VNTRs), are present in all human beings but that they varied and this variation could be used to establish the identity of a person and he named his technique Genetic Fingerprinting.
- Best Test for Paternity (cf. for Identification best is Fingerprinting) Living.
- Ideal Sample Blood (WBCs).
- Most common sample: Buccal Smear Dead. Ideal Sample **Spleen*** and Brain (After PCR technique, this concept is less relevant).
- Preservative: **EDTA**/Temperature of **specimen -20 degree Celsius***.

Six Steps to Obtain a DNA Fingerprint:

1. Extracting the DNA.
2. Cutting or amplifying the DNA
3. Separating the fragments with electrophoresis.
4. Transferring the fragments to a nylon membrane (**Southern Blot Test**).
5. Tagging the fragments with a DNA probe.
6. Visualizing the fragments through autoradiography.

Potential Question Zone

Northern Blotting is a method designed to detect a specific RNA sequence or **mRNA** sequence. Developed by Alwine, Kemp, and Stark. (Memorizer→ **rN(orth)A**)

Western Blotting: Method of detecting a specific protein from a protein mixture. Introduced by Towbin. Detection of **anti-HIV antibodies** in a human serum

Southern Blotting: Developed by E. M. Southern for the identification of a specific **DNA** sequence from a DNA sample
(Memo→**DNA-Dakshin**)

In Praise of Mitochondrial DNA (Non-nuclear DNA)

- Passes from generation to generation by the **maternal lineage (from mothers only)– Siblings have identical mitochondrial DNA.**
- Mutates rarely.
- When nuclear DNA doesn't exist (e.g., hair has no nuclear DNA, the dead may contain mitoDNA).
- Tenacious (survive in old Bones and Teeth).

MCQs

1. **If the father has blood group genotype AO and the mother's blood group genotype BO. The offspring may have blood group genotype:**
   A. A
   B. B
   C. AB
   D. All of the above

2. **In old blood stained fibre, blood grouping is done by:**
   A. Benzidine test
   B. Absorption elution test
   C. Precipitin test
   D. Hemin crystal test

3. **Which of the following sign will indicate that menstrual blood was antemortem?**
   A. Alkaline
   B. Light pink
   C. Does not clot unless mixed with seminal fluid
   D. Shows endometrial and vaginal cells

4. **Takayama reagent is used in:**
   A. Guiacum test
   B. Castle mayer test
   C. Haemin crystal test
   D. Haemochromogen test

5. **Which is a wrong match?**

Test for blood stain	*Positive colour*
A. Benzedine test	Blue
B. Guiacum test	Deep blue
C. Castle mayer test	Pink purple
D. Leucomalachite test	Pink

1 D **2** B **3** C **4** D **5** D

6. **In leucomaiachite test, the positive test is indicated by ..... colour.**
   A. Peacock blue
   B. Deep purple
   C. Red
   D. *Khaki*

7. **Best method to prove paternity is:**
   A. Blood grouping
   B. Fingerprints
   C. Phenotypic resemblance
   D. DNA fingerprinting

8. **In Takayama test, which of the following is seen under microscope?**
   A. Yellowish to brownish rhomboid crystals
   B. Yellow needle shaped crystals
   C. Pink feathery structures
   D. Spherical granules

9. **Which is the best to determine paternity?**
   A. Fingerprinting
   B. DNA fingerprinting
   C. Blood group
   D. HLA

10. **Species identification is done by:**
    A. Neutron activation analysis (N.A.A.)
    B. Precipitin test
    C. Benzidine test
    D. Spectroscopy

6 A 7 D 8 C 9 B 10 B

11
Impotence, Sterility and MTP

- **Impotence** is the inability of a person to perform sexual intercourse. Impotence cannot be placed as a defence for rape.
- **Sterility** is the inability of the male to beget children and in the female, the inability to conceive children.
- **Frigidity** is the inability to start or maintain the sexual arousal pattern in the female.
- The question of impotence and sterility may arise in:

  Civil
  - Nullity of marriage
  - Divorce
  - Adultery
  - Disputed paternity and legitimacy
  - Suits of adoption.

  Criminal*
  - Adultery
  - Rape
  - Unnatural offences.
- **Quod Hanc (literal Latin Translation:** Impotence because of this) a person may show psychic impotence with one woman but can perform the sexual act successfully with another woman. It is found that some persons are *impotent* with regard to their spouses, but potent as to others — this is called ***impotency quod hanc***.
- **Vaginismus** is involuntary spasm of perineal muscle so that sexual intercourse is not possible.

Treatment is psychotherapy.

- After vasectomy, the person should be advised to abstain from sexual intercourse for about **3 months.**

ARTIFICIAL INSEMINATION

- It is artificial introduction of semen into the vagina cervix or uterus to produce pregnancy.
- One ml. of semen is deposited by means of syringe in or near cervix.

Indications

- When the husband is impotent.
- When the husband is unable to deposit the semen in vagina due to hypospadias.
- When the husband is sterile.
- When there is Rh-incompatibility between husband and wife.
- When husband is suffering from hereditary disease.

Legal Problems of Artificial Insemination

- **Adultery** – Donor and recipient cannot be held guilty of adultery in India under Sec. 497 IPC.
- **Legitimacy** – Such a child is illegitimate, if the sperm is from sperm bank and the child needs to be adopted legally.
- **Consent** of both husband and wife is required for receiving artificial insemination, and also consent of donor and his wife are necessary.
- If A.I. is due to impotence and not sterility it can be a ground for **divorce.**
- If A.I. is without consent of husband, he can sue for divorce.

Test Tube Baby

- The ovum is removed from the ovary of the woman and is fertilized outside the body. At the stage

Blastocyst*, the embryo is returned to the uterus, which gets implanted in the endometrium.

Surrogate Birth

- Artificial insemination with the semen of the barren woman's husband is carried out in a hired woman.
- In 2008, the Supreme Court in the Baby Manji's case (Japanese Baby) has held that **commercial surrogacy is permitted in India.**

Suppositious Child: It's a fictitious child. Never born by the woman but there is a false claim that the child belongs to her.

Conclusive proof of legitimacy—Any person was born during the continuance of a valid marriage between his mother and any man, or within **280 days after its dissolution**, the mother remaining unmarried, shall be conclusive proof **(Sec. 112 IEA).**

Memorizer → **1+1**= 3! How? [**2+legitimate child**].

POTENTIAL QUESTIONS ZONE

Assisted Reproductive Technologies (ART) Regulation Bill

The Union Health Ministry has passed the Assisted Reproductive Technologies (ART) regulation bill. According to the bill, anyone acting as a surrogate mother should be between **21-35 years** and cannot give birth **to more than five children** (including her own). The bill has now been sent to the law ministry.

The bill comprises some landmark stipulations:

- Surrogate mothers are not allowed to undertake embryo transfer for the same parents over **three times.**
- To have a married woman as a surrogate mother, **her spouse's consent is obligatory**.
- Only an **Indian citizen** can be considered for surrogacy within India and women cannot be sent abroad for surrogacy.

Contd.

Contd.

- The donor's identity has to be kept **strictly confidential**.
- A prospective surrogate mother should not engage in any act that may harm foetus during the pregnancy period or after birth.
- The **baby's birth certificate** should bear the name of **those individuals who** had **commissioned** the surrogacy.
- In case of any congenital abnormality, the commissioning parents would have to take the child's custody.

VIRGINITY AND PREGNANCY

- **A True Virgin** is a female who has not experienced sexual intercourse, vagina is tight and narrow, hymen may or may not show rupture.
  A FalseVirgin→Hymen intact but experienced sexual intercourse. **Labia minora is cutaneous*** and labia majora is fleshy and lax.
- Defloration means loss of virginity.
  - Tears on hymen caused by sexual intercourse or by foreign body is situated posterolaterally, i.e., 5 or 7 O' clock position.
  - Fimbriated hymen→looks like torn hymen.
  - Tears on hymem caused by **masturbation** is situated anterolaterally, i.e., between 11 and 1 O'clock.
  - **Glaister-keen Rod** used to grade tear of hymen.
- **Causes of rupture of hymen:**
  - An accident—Hymen does not rupture by riding, jumping, dancing etc.
  - Masturbation.
  - **Solapith a weed introduced into vagina can result in rupture.**

ABORTION

MTP Act

- The Medical Termination of Pregnancy Act was passed in 1971.
- Indications of MTP are: **"SETH"**.

Social:
Failure of contraceptive methods in case of a **married**** woman.

Eugenic:
Child born with serious physical or mental abnormalities.

Therapeutic:
Continuation of pregnancy endangers life.

Humanitarian:
Rape resulting in pregnancy.

- **Consent of husband is not necessary. (cf. *Sterilization where both couple consent required*).**
- The age of woman for abortion is over 18 years.
- MTP Act, 1971 allows termination of pregnancy upto 20 weeks.
- If the period of pregnancy is below 12 weeks, it can be terminated by a single doctor.
- If the period of pregnancy is between 12 and 20 weeks, two doctors must concur that there is an indication.

Qualification

For termination up to 20 weeks:
RMP + degree/diploma in Obs and Gynae.
For termination up to 12 weeks:

- RMP with 6 months junior residency in Obs and Gynae.
- RMP with experience of 25 cases (at least 5 done independently).

Consent in MTP

- If married—her own written consent. Husband's consent not needed.
- If unmarried and above 18 years—her own written consent.
- If below 18 years—written consent of her guardian.
- If mentally unstable—written consent of her guardian.

Methods of Criminal Abortion

Abortifacient Drugs

- **Ecbolics**
  - They increase uterine contractions.
  - Ergot is the most commonly used ecbolic.
- **Emmenagogues**
  - They increase the menstrual flow.
  - Sanguinarin, estrogens, senecio are chief emmenagogues.

Other Methods

- **Syringing**

  Salt Poisoning Abortion
  - A syringe of a concentrated salt solution is injected into the amniotic fluid. The foetus then breathes and swallows the hyper-salted amniotic fluid.
  - This abortion procedure was first developed in Nazi concentration camps.
  - Used after 16 weeks, cost effectiveness and ease of administration.
- Rupture of membranes.
- Dilatation of cervix.
- **Cupping:**
  - Practised in advanced pregnancy.
  - It results in placental separation.
- **Abortion sticks:** Calotropis, Plumbago Rosea, Zeylancia, Nerium Odorum is used as—abortion stick.

Medicolegal Aspect of Pregnancy

I. **Concealed pregnancy** before marriage a valid ground for **divorce.**

   Duration of pregnancy assumes importance when legitimacy of a **posthumous child** (***after death of biological father***) is questioned.

II. **False Pregnancy: Pseudocyesis/Phantom/ Hysterical.**

Woman feigning pregnancy
- To avoid capital punishment (**Sec. 416 Cr.P.C** – Woman sentenced to death is found to be pregnant).
- Compel a person to marriage.
- Secure more maintenance in case of divorce.

III. Multiple Pregnancies

Hellin's Law deals with multiple pregnancies.

A. **Superfe-C-undation**–Fertilization of two different ova released in the same **One cycle** (**Memorizer**→One **C** One **Cycle** 2 Ovas).

B. **Superfetation**–Fertilization of two ova released in different cycles.

Miscarriage

• **Sec 312 IPC** does not permit any person including the pregnant woman to miscarry (even **with consent**).
• **Sec 313 IPC** is miscarriage→ **against the consent** of the pregnant woman (cognizable, non-bailable, non-compoundable).
• **Sec 314 IPC** Death of woman caused by act done with intent to cause miscarriage.
• **Sec 315 IPC** Act done with intent to prevent child being born alive or to cause it to die after birth.
• **Sec 316 IPC** Causing death of **Quick** unborn child by act amounting to **Culpable homicide.** **(Memorizer→ Six : Quick –Fix)**

MCQs

1. **Opinion in a male with normal genitalia, about potency is worded as:**
   A. Person is potent
   B. The individual is not impotent
   C. The individual is capable of sexual act
   D. There is nothing to suggest that the person is not capable of sexual intercourse
2. **Quoad is an individual who is:**
   A. Impotent
   B. Potent
   C. Impotent only for particular woman
   D. Became potent after surgery
3. **Precocious puberty is caused by:**
   A. Adrenal tumors
   B. Thyroid dysfunction
   C. Pituitary tumors
   D. Tumors of cerebellum
4. **A female may become sterile with occupational exposure to:**
   A. Mercury **B.** Lead
   C. Aluminium **D.** Asbestos
5. **In fimbriate hymen notches are:**
   A. Mostly asymmetrical
   B. Located anteriorly
   C. Not covered with mucous membrane
   D. Extending to the vaginal wall
6. **Tears in hymen from sexual act are mostly seen at:**
   A. 12 O'clock position
   B. 3 O'clock position
   C. 5 O'clock position
   D. 10 O'clock position

1 D **2** C **3** A **4** B **5** B **6** C

7. Presence of carunculae myrtiformes indicate:
A. Virginity
B. Defloration
C. Previous surgical procedure
D. Previous child birth

8. Premature expulsion of products of conception any time before full term is known legally as:
A. Still birth
B. Premature birth
C. Abortion
D. Miscarriage

9. Abortions are more common during:
A. 1st trimester
B. 2nd trimester
C. 3rd trimester
D. Any time

10. Commonly used substance for criminal abortion is:
A. Ergot
B. Marking nut
C. Quinine
D. Lead compounds

11. Cause of abortion in cupping is:
A. Rupture of membranes
B. Placental separation
C. Increased uterine contractions
D. Increased menstrual flow

12. Medical termination of pregnancy by a single doctor can be undertaken upto:
A. 8 weeks
B. 12 weeks
C. 16 weeks
D. 20 weeks

13. For medical termination of pregnancy, consent is required from:
A. Husband of the lady
B. Both husband and wife
C. Concerned lady
D. Guardian

14. The MTP Act was introduced in:
A. 1961
B. 1971
C. 1974
D. 1975

---

7 D 8 C 9 A 10 A 11 B 12 B 13 C 14 B

15. The feminine of impotence is:

A. Rigidity
B. Frigidity
C. Sterility
D. Flaccidity
E. Nymphomania

16. The most common maternal cause of abortion is:

A. Tuberculosis
B. Syphilis
C. General debility
D. Sexual weakness

17. Impotence may be pleaded as a ground for all *except:*

A. Divorce
B. Rape
C. Adultery
D. Unnatural sexual offence

18. The most striking symptom of pregnancy is:

A. Enlargement of abdomen
B. Morning sickness
C. Frequency of micturition
D. Cessation of menstruation

19. Hymen can be ruptured by:

A. Solapith
B. Mastrubation
C. Sanitary tampons
D. Horse riding
E. Any of the above

20. All the following are indications for doing Medical Termination of Pregnancy *except:*

A. Pregnancy from rape
B. Substantial risk of delivering seriously handicapped baby
C. Very poor socio-economic position of the family
D. Injury to physical and mental health of the pregnant woman

15 B **16** B **17** B **18** D **19** E **20** C

21. The most important sign of defloration is:
A. Enlarged nipple
B. Dilation of vaginal canal
C. Enlarged breasts
D. Ruptured hymen

22. Weight of the normal uterus is:
A. 30-45 gm B. 45-60 gm
C. 60-70 gm D. 80-100 gm

23. Hegar's sign is for the detection of:
A. Dead foetus B. Virginity
C. Sterility D. None of the above

24. The most important cause of temporary impotence is:
A. Over excitement B. Guilt
C. Fear D. Aversion

25. All the following could be seen in a false virgin *except:*
A. Flabby breasts
B. Tight and narrow vagina
C. Labia separated
D. Thick and elastic injured hymen

26. The minimum age for medical termination of pregnancy is:
A. 16 years B. 18 years
C. 20 years D. 24 years

27. Both mother and father have AB blood group, blood group in children can be:
A. A only
B. A and AB only
C. B and AB only
D. A, B or AB

28. Legally "Abortion" is termination of pregnancy:
A. Before 6 weeks B. Before 16 weeks
C. Before 26 weeks D. Before full term

---

21 D 22 C 23 D 24 C 25 B 26 B 27 D 28 D

12

Toxicology

Toxicology

1. Forensic toxicology—medical and legal aspects of harmful effects of chemicals on human being.
2. Clinical toxicology—disease caused in human being on exposure to chemical substances.

Toxinology: Substance produced by living organisms, which are dangerous to man.

Paracelsus – Father of (ancient) Toxicology.

Paracelsus's Three Laws of Toxicology

1. The dose makes the poison.
2. Specificity of toxic effects are due to the unique chemical structure.
3. Humans are animals; therefore, the study of animals can provide useful insight.

Orfila–Father of (modern) Toxicology.

Descending Order of Lethality

Botulinus toxin > Strychnine > Arsenic > Cyanide >Thallium

Botulinum Toxin's Killing Style*: It irreversibly binds to cholinergic nerve terminals and **stops acetylcholine release** from the axon. Most lethal toxin.

Ideal Homicidal Poison

- Most important characteristic features of ideal homicidal poison are:

- It should cause a slow and gradual death.
- It should resemble some natural condition.

Some common poisons and the disease they resembles:

Poisons	*Disease*
1. Arsenic	• Cholera • Fading Measles • Addison's Disease
2. Strychnine	• Tetanus
3. Zinc	• Malarial Chills
4. **Thallium**	• **Natural Death** • **Guillain-Barré syndrome** • **Porphyria**
5. Di-nitro compounds	• Thyrotoxicosis
6. Organophosphates	• Bronchial Asthma
7. Bromides	• Acne

- **Thallium** is an ideal homicidal poison.The **triad** of gastroenteritis, polyneuritis and hair loss is a strong indicator of thallium poisoning. Heart may show fatty degeneration (**tabby cat striations**). **Signe de sourcil** is a French term for "The eyebrow sign". The outer 2/3rd of eyebrow falls characteristic of Thallium Poisoning.

Ideal Suicidal Poison

- **Characters:** Cheap, easily available, highly toxic, tasteless or of pleasant taste. Capable of producing painless death.
- **Cyanide** is ideal suicidal poison*.
- Organophosphorus compounds are most commonly used as suicidal poison.

Stupefying Agents

- Dhatura, Cannabis indica, Chloral Hydrate also known as **Dry Wine** (Strong in taste, pungent odor).

Abortifacient Drugs

- Calotropis, oleanders, aconite, ergot, lead etc.

Cattle Poisoning

- The usual poisons are ***abrus precatorious,*** oleanders calotropis, aconite, arsenic, organophosphorus, strychnine, zinc phosphide, nitrate etc.

Arrow Poisons

- Abrus precatorius, croton oil, calotropis, aconite strychnine, curare and snake venom.

Occupational Poisonous Substance

Cyanides	Jewellery and electroplating
Carbon monoxide	Steel blast furnaces
Carbon disulphide	Explosives, paint rayon
Hydrogen sulphide	Tanneries, oil wells, paper making.

Household Poisons

- Nail polish remover – Acetone
- Marking ink – Aniline
- Ink remover –
    - Oxalic acid
    - Na hypo chloride 5%

Sweet Poisons

i. Aconite.
ii. Lead acetate.
iii. Glycols.
iv. Methyl salicylate.
v. Bromoform.

Forensic Toxicology

Poisons Act	1919
Dangerous Drugs Act	1930
Drugs and Cosmetics Act	1940

- Main Aim – Control quality, purity and strength of drugs*.

- Ayurveda and Unani medicines included in 1964 Amendments.
- Label should display formula ingredients of medical formulation.

Drugs and Cosmetics Rule	1945
Pharmacy Act	1948
Drugs Control Act	1950
Drugs and Magic Remedies (Objectionable Advertisement) Act	1954
Opium Act	1957
Opium Act	1978

Narcotic Drugs and Psychotropic Substance Act*1985

(**Memorizer**→NARCO has **5** letters not 6, so 8**5**)

[Recommends treatment and rehab of users. Punishment for drug peddlers]

Narcotics: COP→(Cocaine, Cannabis, Opium, Poppy)

Psychotropics (LSD, Amphetamines etc.)

Alchohol, Paracetamol, Nicotine is NOT included in NDPS Act*.

Prevention of illicit traffic* in Narcotic drugs and PSA	1988

Drugs and Cosmetics Rules, 1945

- Framed under: Drugs Act, 1940.
- **Classification of drugs in schedules:**
  - C–Biological and special products.
  - E–Poisons.
  - **F**–Vaccines and sera [**V**accines Stored in **F**ridge].
  - **G**–**H**ormonal preparations **[G-H]**.
  - H–drugs/poisons to be sold on prescription of RMP [**H**andwriting of Doctor's **P**rescription].
  - J–Diseases for cure of which no drug should be advertised.
  - L–Antibodies, Antihistaminic, chemotherapeutic agents.
  - X–Potential drug of abuse.

Sections of law pertaining of Poisons/Poisoning

39 CrPC	Information to police/magistrate
175 CrPC	Investigation
176 IPC	Punishment for noncompliance (6 months/1000 Rs)
193 IPC	Punishment for false evidence (3-7 years and fine)
202 IPC	Punishment for concealing information (6 months/fine)
284 IPC	Negligent conduct with respect to poisonous substance Term max. of 6 months, or fine Rs. 1000 or both
299 IPC	Culpable homicide
300 IPC	Murder
304A IPC	Causing death by negligence Term of max. 2 years or fine or both
309 IPC	Attempt to commit suicide (1 year/fine)
324 IPC	Voluntarily causing hurt by dangerous weapons or means Term max. 3 years or fine or both
326 IPC	Voluntarily causing grievous hurt by dangerous weapons or means Imprisonment for life or Term up to ten years and also fine
328 IPC	Causing hurt by means of poison etc with intent to commit an offence Term up to 10 years and also fine

General Management of Poisoning are:

i. Stabilization.
ii. Gut decontamination.
iii. Antidote administration.
iv. Elimination.
v. Symptomatic treatment.

1. *Stabilization:*
   - **Scandinavian Regime*** is a term used for anti-shock measures when the patient is going into shock. It includes A B C D E of resuscitation.

     A—Airways
     B—Breathing
     C—Circulation
     D—Drugs
     E—Evaluation

2. *Gut Decontamination*:

The various methods to remove poison from GIT are:

- Emesis.
- Gastric lavage.
- Catharsis.
- Activated charcoal.
- Whole bowel irrigation.
- *Emesis.*
  - Best method to induce emesis is by inducing GAG REFLEX*/hypertonic saline.
  - **IPECACUANHA** is the only pharmaceutical agent recommended to induce vomitting.
- *Gastric lavage*

The tube	(Ewald or Boas tube)	
Diameter	1 cm	
Length	1 and ½ meter	
Mark at	50 cm	
Openings	Lateral	
Patient position	Left lateral or prone	
Material	Potassium permanganate	1 : 5000
	Sodium bicarbonate	5%
	Tannic acid	4%
	Sodium or potassium iodide	1%
	Calcium lactate	1–3%
	Saturated lime water or starch	

- *Contraindication for gastric lavage is* **[Memorizer→ sound of 'Ka']**
  1. **K**Corrosives (Absolute contraindication except carbolic acid).
  2. **K**Convulsants/CNS stimulants use with precaution.
  3. **K**Comatose patient.
  4. Volatile poison. **K**(C)erosine
  5. Upper GI pathology (Esophageal varices).
  6. Hypothermic patient (**K**Cold).
  7. Severe heart disease.
  8. Advanced pregnancy.

- Gastric lavage is useful within **3 hours** of ingestion of poison.
- Water or normal saline is the **most commonly*** used solution for gastric lavage.
- $KMnO_4$
  - ♦ It is used for oxidisable poisons.
  - ♦ In opium poisoning* $KMnO_4$ is used in higher concentrations.
  - ♦ In opium poisoning* Gastric lavage is done even when opium has been administered through parenteral route.
  - ♦ $KMnO_4$ is not useful in heavy metal poisoning.

Heavy metals	*Substance used for gastric lavage*
Arsenic	Freshly prepared Ferric Oxide (Hydrated)
Mercury	Sodium Formaldehyde Sulphoxylate
Copper	Potassium Ferrocyanide (Non-toxic salt of cyanosis)
Iron	Desferrioxamine

  - ♦ Calcium gluconate is used in oxalates.
  - ♦ Sodium thiosulphate is used in cyanides.

- *Catharsis*
  - **Sorbitol (D-glucitol)*** is the cathartic of choice in adults.
- *Activated Charcoal*
  - Charcoal is activated by using steam, carbon monoxide etc.
  - Charcoal acts by **AD**sorption* (not by Absorption).

Potential Question Zone (PQZ) wrt. Charcoal (Memorizer→Char – BAARbiCHurate)	
Indications	*Contraindications*
Barbiturates	
Tylenol	Caustics
Anticholinergics	Hydrocarbons (and most water soluble compounds)
Carbamazepine	**Heavy Metals, Cyanide***
Ibuprofen	Alcohol
Phenothiazines	Lithium
Salicylates, TCAs	Phosphorus
Theophyline	
Clonidine	

3. *Antidote Administration:*

Poisons	*Antidotes*
1. Paracetamol	• Acetyl cysteine • Methionine*
2. Methanol, Ethylene Glycol	• 4-Methyl Pyrozole (fomipazole) [competitive inhibitor of Alcohol Dehydrogenase] • Ethyl alcohol
3. Benzodiazepinus	Flumazenil
4. Opiates	Nalaxone
5. Organophosphates	• Atropine • Oximes (P.A.M., D.A.M etc)
6. *Dhatura*	Physostigmine
7. Botulinum toxin	Guanidine
8. Cyanide	• Para-Amino-Propiophenone (4-PAPP) • Dicobalt acetate • Vitamin B_{12} (Hydroxy cobalamine) • 4-Dimethyl amino phenol (4-DAMP) • Amyl Nitrite + Na Thiosulphate
9. Methemoglobinemia	Methylene blue
10. Thallium	Prussian blue (K Hexa Cyanoferrate)
11. Carbon monoxide	• Vitamin E (Tocopherol) • *Hyper Baric Oxygen*

[**N.B.**→$CuSO_4$ Copper Sulphate is a poison and also antidote for Phosphorous].

Chemical Antidotes

Common salt	Silver nitrate
Albumen	Mercury chloride
Dialyzed iron	Arsenic
Copper sulphate	Phosphorous

1. *BAL*
   - British antilewisite or Dimercarpol.
   - It is given by intramuscular route*.
   - Contraindicated in
     - Liver damage
     - G6PD deficiency
     - Iron and cadmium toxicity*.
2. *EDTA* is contraindicated in mercury*.
3. *Pencillamine* is contraindicated in Arsenic*.
4. *Desferoxamine* is also useful in treatment of toxicity with radioactive heavy metals.*

Universal Antidote: It is combination of physical and chemical antidotes.

Magnesium oxide (1 part) neutralizes acid without gas formation.

Charcoal (2 parts) absorbs alkaloids.

Tannic acid (1 part) precipitates alkaloids.

Coma Cocktail:

Combination of 3 medicines can be given in unknown poisoning with coma [remember **DNB**].

Dextrose (50%) 100 ml.

Nalaxone 2 mg.

B_1 (Thiamine) 100 mg.

4. *Elimination:*

Forced Diuresis

Saline Diuresis	*Alkaline Diuresis*	*Acid Diuresis*
Alcohols	Chlorphenoxyacetic acid herbicides	**Amphetamines**
Bromide	Chlorpropamide	**Chloroquine**
Calcium	Diflusinal	Cocaine
Fluoride	Fluoride	Local anaesthetics
Lithium	Methotrexate	**Phencyclidine**
Meprobamate	Phenobarbital	Quinidines
Potassium	Sulfonamides	Quinine
Isoniazid	Salcylates	Sympathomimetics
		TCAs
		Tocainide

Hemodialysis

Hemodialysis is useful in:

B—Barbiturates, Bromides, **Boric Acid (Boiled Lobster Appearance)***

L—Lithium

A—Alcohol

(Methanol–*absolutely indicated*[NEET], glycols)*

S—Salicylates

T—Theophylline, Thiocyanates

[***PQZ→Boiled Lobster Appearance and Boric Acid:**

In severe poisonings, a beefy red skin rash, affecting palms, soles, buttocks and scrotum, characterized as a **"boiled lobster appearance"**. The intense erythema is followed by extensive exfoliation. D/d Staphylococcal scalded Skin Syndrome.

Reversible alopecia has been reported following exposure to Boric acid].

Haemodialysis is not done in:

- Benzodiazepines
- Chloroquine; **Copper sulphate**
- **Digitalis**
- Heroin
- Kerosene
- Organophosphates.

Hemoperfusion

Hemoperfusion is useful in:

- Chloramphenicol
- Disopyramide
- Charcoal hemoperfusion is used in **Hypnotic–sedatives [Barbiturates]***
  - Ethchlorvynol
  - Glutethimide
  - Meprobamate
  - Methaqualone
- Phenytoin
- Procainamide
- Theophylline.

Peritoneal Dialysis cffectively removes:

- Alcohol
- Long acting barbiturates
- Chloral hydrate
- Lithium
- Salicylates
- Sodium chlorate.

Exchange Transfusion

- Adv. of Exchange transfusion removes poison affecting RBCs (as in Methemoglobinemia or arsenic induced hemolysis).

5. *Symptomatic Treatment.*

PRESERVATIVES, PRESERVATION AND PRESERVED

Preservation of Viscera

1. Stomach and its contents.
2. 30 cm small interline and contents.
3. Liver > 500 gms.
4. One kidney/Half of each.
5. Blood 100 cc (in NaF), Minimum 10 ml*.
   - Blood best specimen.
     NaF
     – Prevents bacterial fermentation.
     – Stops the spontaneous hydrolysis of poisons.
     – Blocks clotting.
   - Peripheral blood concentration (**femoral vein**) have been shown to be more reliable (because of redistribution) for toxicological analysis than the conventional heart blood.

PQZ : IPC - 201 [Memorizer→T(w)O (n0t) preserve ONE's v1scera] Failure to Preserve Viscera
The prosector is supposed to preserve the viscera till IO collects it or authorizes the prosector to destroy the material. If the prosector destroys the viscera without permission of IO, he is likely to be charged and punished under IPC section 201 for causing loss of evidence.

6. Urine > 100 cc–(in Thymol)* [Toulene* is the best preservative for urine examination]
   - The best preservative for preservation of viscera is rectified spirit.
   - Most commonly used preservative is saturated sodium chloride.
   - While despatching blood and urine for chemical analysis **Sodium Fluoride** is added as preservative in **50 mg/10 ml** concentration.
   - Viscera is stored at 4°C.
   - Histopathology specimen is preserved in 10% neutral formalin/95% Alcohol.
   - Virology specimen 50% glycerol in buffer saline.
   - Rectified spirit is not used in:
     - Alcohol
     - Phenol
     - Phosphorous
       [Alcohol cannot be used, because alcohol prevents the luminosity of phosphorus in dark.]
     - Paraldehyde.
   - Formaldehyde is used for preservation of Museum specimens and not for preservation of viscera for toxicological analysis.
   - Formalin is 40% formaldehyde.
   - NaF should be added to urine, blood, vitrous humor for alcohol estimation and to samples of:
     - Cocaine (C).
     - Carbon monoxide (C)→3C's.
     - Cyanide (C).

Special Preservations

- Liver is the **most important tissue** because it concentrates many substances.
- Heart–Strychnine, digitalis.
- Spleen–It is the best organ for cyanide poisoning (best specimen for DNA analysis).

- Brain–Alkaloids, organophosphates, volatile organic poisons.
- Bile–Narcotic drugs, cocaine, methadone, glutathione, barbiturates, tranquillizers, opiates and acetaminophen.
- Vitreous–Alcohol, chloroform [Vitreous humour is preserved by keeping at 4ºC for 48 hours, normally preservative is of no value. Vitreous humour alcohol concentrations are a little higher than blood. Though could be preserved with sodium fluoride (10 mg/ml)].
- Lung–Gaseous poison, HCN, alcohol, chloroform.
- Bone–Arsenic, antimony, thallium, radium.
- Skin–C/o hypodermic injections (10 cm radius about site with muscle and fat), snake bite.
- Hair, nails, uterus, spinal cord–When indicated.
- CSF–(in 10 mg NaF/ml of fluid) in alcohol intoxication.
- Body fat—Endrin, DDT (Organo Chlorines).
- Muscle–When internal organs badly putrified. Skeletal muscle of buttock best specimen for toxicology in embalming.

I. Screening Tests (Qualitiative)

Immunoassays: Most commonly used drug screening tests.

Immunoassays	*True*	*False*
Positive	Test correctly detects Poison/drug	Test incorrectly detects when no Poison/drug
Negative	Test correctly confirms the absence of Poison/drug	Test fails to detect the presence of Poison/drug

II. **Confirmatory Test:** Mass Spectrometry (MS).

III. **Chromatography:** Analytical procedure used for **Separation** of poisons/drugs.

(a) High performance liquid chromatography (HPLC).

(b) Gas chromatography (GC).

Chromatography is a definitive technique to establish structure of poison*.

Coloration of Postmortem Staining

• Dark brown/yellow	Phosphorus
• Brick red	Hydrocyanic acid
• Cherry red	Carbon monoxide
• Chocolate color	Chlorate of potash
• Dark brown (Chocolate Cyanosis)	Aniline, *Nitrites*, Nitroglycerine, *spirits* of Niter
• Bluish-green	Hydrogen sulphide
• Bronze colour	Clostridium perfringens
• Black colour	Opiates
• Blue skin	Gadolinium

Smells of Different Poisonings (Cranial Cavity is opened first to differentiate smells).

- Garlic–Salicylate, Phosphorus, Arsenic. Al–phosphide (Celphos).
- Bitter almonds–Cyanide poisoning (HCN), prussic acid.
- Sewer gas smell–H_2S.
- Kerosene odour–Organophosphates.
- Smell of burnt rope–Cannabis.(AIIMS–May 2014)
- Sweet and fruity–Ethanol, methanol, chloroform.
- Acrid/Pear–Chloral hydrate, paraldehyde.
- Shoe polish–Nitrobenzene.
- Hospital odour–Carbolic acid.
- Rotten eggs–Disulfiram, H_2S.
- Rotten fish–Aniline.

[N.B. 'The Nose Knows Box'→Chap. 17]

Radiopaque Densities (Abdominal X-rays)
Chloral hydrate coated pills
Calcium
Heavy metals
Lithium
Phenothiazines
Salicylates

Causes of Anion Gap
A normal AG has been defined as 12 G +/- 4 mEq/L Methanol, Ethanol Ethylene glycol, Phenols Uremia Iron, INH Lactate Salicylates

Effect of poison on pupil

Miosis	*Mydriasis*	*Nystagmus*
Mitotic (Pilocarpine) Opiates Pontine hemorrhage Organophosphates	Dhatura, Chlorinated hydrocarbons [Endrin[NEET], aldrin, DDT, BHC, toxaphene, strobane]	• Anticonvulsants (phenytoin, carbamazepine, valproic acid, lamotrigine, topiramate) • Ethanol • Lithium • Dextromethorphan • Phencyclidine (PCP) • Ketamine • Lysergic acid diethylamide (LSD)

[PQZ→**Cornpicker's Pupil**–Unilateral Mydriasis by Pollens]

Causes of Diaphoretic Skin
Sympathomimetics • Amphetamine • Cocaine • LSD Organophosphates Aspirin PCP

Autopsy Changes in Certain Poisoning

- Chalky white teeth→Sulphuric acid.
- Black tongue and teeth→Cocaine.
- **Stomach**
  - Bloating Paper Appearance→Sulphuric Acid.
  - Leathery Mucosa of Stomach→Carbolic Acid.
  - **R**ed Velvet Mucosa→a**Rsenic.**

Coloration of mucous membrane of stomach

Green	Ferrous sulphate
Blue	Amytal
Pink	Soneryl
Slate	Mercury
White particulate	Arsenic
Black	Sulphuric acid, Acetic acid, Hydrochloric acid
Yellow	Nitric acid
Buffed white	Carbolic acid
Brown	Cresols
Blue/Green	Copper
Grey white/yellow	Phosphorus

- **Intestine**
  Multiple patchy haemorrhages→Mercury.
- **Kidney.**

Poisons Causing Necrosis of Proximal Convoluted Tubule

- Mercuric chloride.
- Lysol.
- Carbon tetrachloride.
- Oxalic acid.
- Phenol.

Heart:

- Arsenic→Subendocardial haemorrhage.
- AL. Phosphide→Subendocardial infarcts. (**N.B.**→Also See Page 384).

Conditions which Delay Putrefaction:

- Carbolic acid.
- Zinc chloride.
- Strychnine.
- Chronic heavy metal poisoning.
- Washing disease.
- Anaemia.

Putrefaction Sets in Rapidly in Cases of:

- Septicemia.
- Peritonitis.
- Inflammatory and septic condition.
- General anasarca.
- Asphyxia.

CORROSIVE POISONS

Mineral Acids

- They produce **coagulation necrosis causing more damage** than irritant poisons.
- **Hygroscopic** extraction of water leading to **cellular dehydration** results in **mucosal erosion**.
- Converts Haemoglobin to Heme/Hematin.
- Results in perforation.
- Nitric acid produces a **yellowish stain**.
- Sulphuric acid and caustic **alkalis reddish-brown** stains.
- Hydrochloric acid and carbolic acid whitish or **greyish yellow stains** on the skin and mucous membranes.
- **Magenstrasse also known as Stomach Street**–Tubular and thicker area of the stomach close to the lesser curvature. Acid Agents flow through this pathway. Damage of stomach due to corrosives depends on whether stomach is full or empty. Greatest damage is along the lesser curvature.
- Food filled Stomach–Damage-Lesser Curvature
- Empty Stomach–Damage-Lower 2/3rd of Stomach.

Sulphuric Acid

- Sulphuric acid is the strongest corrosive poison.
- Brown to black streaks from angle of mouth present.
- **Blotting paper appearance*** of mucosa of stomach is seen in **H_2SO_4 poisoning.**
- The vomit is brown or black, mucoid, strongly acid and may contain shreds of charred wall of the stomach.
- **Teeth are chalky-white.*** Tounge is swollen, sodden and black.
- Constipation is severe and there is **tenesmus.**
- Edema, erythema and ulceration of the esophagus may be followed by **fibrosis with stricture*** formation and obstruction of the gastric outlet.

- *Fatal dose*–5 to 10 ml.
- *Fatal period*–18 to 24 hours.
- *Causes of death*
  i. Circulatory collapse.
  ii. Spasm or oedema of glottis.
  iii. Collapse due to perforation of stomach.
  iv. Toxaemia.
  v. Delayed death may occur due to hypostatic, pneumonia, secondary infection, renal failure or starvation due to stricture of oesophagus.
- *Treatment:*
  1. Gastric lavage or emetics are **contraindicated**.
  2. The acid should be immediately diluted and neutralised by giving 250 ml of water or milk mixed with 4 tsf. **Of calcium or magnesium oxide (antidote),** aluminium hydroxide gel or calcined magnesia or soap water may be used.
  3. Alkaline carbonates and **bicarbonates, are contraindicated in treatment of H_2SO_4 poisoning because it liberates carbon dioxide, should not be used as they cause gastric dilatation and sometimes rupture**.
  4. Give a demulcent-olive oil, milk, egg-whites, starch water, mineral oil, melted butter.
  5. Prednisolone 60 mg/day may be given to prevent oesophageal stricture and for shock. Later, half an inch diameter of mercury-filled bougie should be passed daily if stricture develops.
  6. Correct shock.
  7. Tracheostomy—If there is edema of the glottis.
  8. Give nothing by mouth.
  9. Skin burns are washed with large amount of water and a paste of magnesium oxide or sodium bicarbonate is applied.

10. Eye burns are irrigated with water or sodium bicarbonate solution for 10 to 15 minutes.
11. Symptomatic.

– *Postmortem appearance*
   i. Corrosion of the mucous membranes of lips, mouth and throat and of the skin over the chin, angles of mouth and hands is seen.
   ii. The necrotic areas are at first greyish-white but soon become brown or black and leathery.

– *Internal*
   i. **Blotting paper appearance** of stomach mucosa (c.f. **Red Velvet mucosa** in Arsenic poisoning).
   ii. The greater part of stomach may be converted into a soft **spongy black mass**, which disintegrates when touched. The stomach wall has a brown or black colour.
   iii. Perforation may occur in sulphuric acid poisoning with the escape of the gastric contents into the peritoneal cavity. Chemical peritonitis and corrosion of organs is seen.

VITRIOLAGE (VITRIOL THROWING)

It comes under Sec. 320 IPC (Grievous hurt/Sixth clause):

- Throwing of sulphuric acid on another individual is known as vitriolage.
- Most common agent used as vitriolage is sulphuric acid.
- Death may result from shock or toxaemia.
- The burns are painless, penetrating and the acid devitalises the tissues and predispose to infection.
- Sometimes, corrosive alkali or juice of marking nut or calotropis is used to disfigure the face.

  – *Treatment*
    ♦ The affected part is washed with plenty of water and soap or sodium or potassium

carbonate. Later, a thick **paste of magnesium oxide or carbonate** is applied.

- The eyes are washed with water and irrigated with a **dilute sodium bicarbonate solution.*** Later a few drops of olive oil or castor oil are put into the eyes.

New Sections for punishing Acid Attack (Memorizer→Acid **3-ew** on a **26 years**)

Sec. 326-A IPC: Voluntarily causing grievous **hurt** by use of acids–**Severe Offence.**

Sec. 326-B IPC: Voluntarily throwing or attempting to throw acid.

NITRIC ACID (HNO_3)

- In concentrated form, it combines with organic matter and produces a yellow discoloration of tissue due to the **production of picric acid (xanthoproteic reaction).**
  - *Signs and symptoms*
    i. They are those of poisoning by sulphuric acid.
    ii. It causes yellow discoloration of the tissues including the crowns of the teeth and yellow stains on the clothing.
    iii. Inhalation of fumes causes lacrimation, photophobia, irritation of air passages and lungs producing sneezing, coughing, dyspnoea and asphyxia.
  - *Fatal dose:* 10 to 15 ml.
  - *Fatal period:* 12 to 24 hours.
  - *Postmortem appearance*
    i. They are those of sulphuric acid but the tissue is stained yellow, except stomach.
    ii. The stomach is soft, friable and ulcerated and brownish discoloration.
    Perforation of stomach is not common.
  - *Treatment*: Same as for sulphuric acid.

Oxalic Acid

- In the form of oxalates, it exists as a natural

constituent of many plants, e.g., **spinach,** rhubarb, cabbage etc.

- It is used **as ink-remover** solution in forgeries.*
  - Action
    - i. Local-corrosive poison. Corrodes mucous membrane of the digestive tract.
    - ii. Systemic
      - a. Shock
      - b. **Hypocalcemia (That's why wall-scrapings and chalk powder can be given as treatment).** Trousseau's Sign[NEET].
      - c. Renal damage.

* Oxalates produce **tubular nephrosis** or necrosis and cause death from **uremia** in 2 to 14 days.

- *Fatal dose:* 15 to 20 gms.
- *Fatal period:* 1 to 2 hrs.
- *Signs and symptoms*
  - ♦ Vomit usually contains altered blood and mucus and has a **'coffee ground' appearance*.**
  - ♦ In oxalic acid poisoning, pulse is feeble and rapid.
  - ♦ If the patient survives for a few hours, **hypocalcemia** and digestive upset occurs.
  - ♦ **Chvostek/Weiss sign:** Carpopedal spasm*, hyperirritability of peripheral nerves.
  - ♦ The urine may be scanty or suppressed and may contain traces of blood, albumin and calcium oxalate crystals.
- *Treatment*

1. The stomach is washed out carefully using **calcium lactate or gluconate**.
2. The antidote for oxalate poisoning is **calcium gluconate 10%,*** 10 ml I.V. at frequent intervals.
3. For oxalate poisoning, any preparation of calcium which converts the poison into

insoluble calcium oxalate are used, e.g., lime water, calcium lactate calcium gluconate, calcium chloride, a suspension of chalk in water or milk.

4. 1.5 gm of chalk will neutralise about one gram of oxalic acid.
5. Parathyroid extract.*
6. Demulcent drinks.

– **Postmortem appearance**

i. Stomach is reddened or eroded or almost **black.***

ii. The stomach contents are gelatinous and **brownish due to acid haematin*** formation.

CARBOLIC ACID

- Carbolic acid is also known as **phenol. Pure form is prismatic 'Needle like Crystals'.**
- Phenol is converted into **hydroquinone and pyrocatechol*** in the body before being excreted in the urine.
  - *Fatal dose*: 1 to 2 gm.
  - *Fatal period:* 3 to 4 hours.
  - *Signs and Symptoms:* Poisoning by carbolic acid is known as carbolism.

Local

a. *Skin*

- It causes burning and numbness due to damage to nerve endings.
- It precipitates protein and coagulates cell contents.
- Produces white opaque eschar.
- Necrosis and gangrene of the tissue, which becomes green white or brown white.

b. *Digestive tract*

- Hot burning pain extends from the mouth to the stomach followed by tingling and later anaesthesia.

c. *Respiratory tract*

- Pulmonary and laryngeal oedema develops due to irritation.

Systemic Effects

- In phenol poisoning, pupils are contracted*.
- Breathing is stertorous.
- Convulsims and lock-jaw occurs.
- Depressant of nervous system, especially the respiratory centre*.
- Headache, giddiness, tinnitus, muscular spasm and later collapse, unconsciousness and coma occur. **Marasmus** is seen in Chronic Phenol Poisoning.
- Urine is scanty and contains albumin and free haemoglobin; suppression may follow.
- ***Carboluria:*** In the body phenol is partially oxidised to **hydroquinone and pyrocatechol** and are excreted in urine along with unchanged phenol. The further oxidation of hydroquinone and pyrocatechol in the urine is the cause of **green*** coloration. This is known as **Carboluria.**

  (**c.f.—Liquid gold*** is a term associated with **Amphetamine Abuse and not Barbiturate**
  Reason: The metabolite of Amphetamine are themselves addictive so people used to sell their urine in weekly market and used to fetch high prices that's how the term **liquid gold** came!! Remember its liquid gold and not golden urine).

  Proximal Tubular Necrosis is seen in Phenol poisoning.
- The hydroquinone and pyrocatechol may cause pigmentation in the cornea and various cartilages– a condition called **Ochronosis.**
  - *Causes of death*
    1. Syncope
    2. Asphyxia due to
       i. Failure of respiration.
       ii. Oedema of glottis.
       iii. Complication, e.g., bronchopneumonia.
  - *Treatment*
    i. The stomach should be washed with plenty of lukewarm water* containing animal

charcoal, olive oil, castor oil, magnesium or sodium sulphate, or saccharated lime with which phenol combines and forms harmless products.

ii. Magnesium sulphate or medicinal liquid paraffins should be left in the stomach.

– **Postmortem appearance**

i. The stomach mucosal folds are swollen and covered by opaque, coagulated, grey or brown mucous membrane. The mucous membrane is thickening and **looks leathery**** (white Leathery appearance).

ii. Liver and spleen–show whitish, hardened patch.

iii. Kidneys–show haemorrhagic nephritis, phenol causes **PCT necrosis.**

– **Key Points**

- Phenol delays putrefaction.
- It causes PCT necrosis.
- It causes leathery appearance of mucosa of stomach.

Carbolic Acid in Urine can be confirmed using– **Benedicts/Fehling's Solution, Ferric Chloride, Bromine Water.**

NON-METALLIC POISONS

Phosphorus

- These are of two varieties:
  - White or crystalline.
  - Red or amorphous.
- It is protoplasmic poison, which affects cellular oxidation.
- Difference between white and red phosphorus is that red phosphorus is non-toxic whereas **whiT*e phosphorus is highly *Toxic (T→Toxic).**

Signs and Symptoms

1. Fulminating Poisoning

- This is seen when more than 1 gm is taken.

- Death usually occurs within 12 hours due to shock.

2. Acute Poisoning

a. *First Stage*
   - Symptoms occur within a few minutes to a few hours and lasts 8 hours to 3 days.
   - Ingestion produces burning pain in the throat and abdomen with intense thirst, nausea, vomiting, diarrhoea and severe abdominal pain.
   - Breath and excreta have **(Garlic like odour)*.**
   - Luminescent vomit and faeces are diagnostic.
   - **Smoking Stool Syndrome*** Faint fumes coming from stools in phosphorus poisoning.
   - Skin contact produces painful penetrating second and third degree burns.

b. *Second Stage*
   - This is a symptom free period lasting for 2-3 days.

c. *Third Stage*
   - Symptom of systemic toxicity.
   - *Fatal dose:* 60-120 mg.
   - *Fatal period*: 2 to 8 days.
   - *Treatment*
     1. Gastric lavage using 1:5000 solution of potassium permanganate oxidises phosphorus into phosphoric acid and phosphates, which are harmless.
     2. **Antidote-copper sulphate:** It coats the particles of phosphorus with a film of copper phosphide which is relatively harmless, ***this antidote is obsolete now.***
     3. **Vitamin K** is useful in treatment (c.f. cyanide treatment vitamin B_{12} is useful).
     4. Oil and fats should be avoided.
     5. Peritoneal or haemodialysis.

6. Burns should be thoroughly washed with 1% copper sulphate solution in water.

- **Postmortem appearances:**
  - In acute poisoning jaundice is produced.
  - The gastric and intestinal contents may smell of garlic.
  - The mucous membranes of the stomach and intestine are yellowish or greyish white in colour.
  - Multiple small or large haemorrhages are seen in the skin, subcutaneous tissues, muscles serosal and mucosal surface.
  - **The liver** becomes swollen, yellow, soft, fatty and is easily ruptured.* After a **week** acute **yellow atrophy appears.***
- **Phossy Jaw (also known as *Glass Jaw**)**
  - ***'Phossy Jaw'***, is osteomyelitis and necrosis of the jaw occurs, with multiple sinuses discharging foul smelling pus.
  - The frequent inhalation of phosphorus fumes over a **period of years** causes necrosis of **the lower jaw** in the region of a decayed tooth.
  - Phossy Jaw was first described by **John Syer Bristo.**
- **Poisoning**

  Phosphorus is known as **Diwali poisons.** Accidental poisoning in children may occur due to chewing of fireworks.

  Diwali Poisons are:
  - Phosphorus.
  - Mercuric cyanide (small tablets when put to flames produce snake like appearance).
  - Antimony.
  - Arsenic.
  - Strontium.

IODINE (PROTOPLASMIC POISON)

- *Action:*
  - It is a protoplasmic poisons fixing protein and causing necrosis.

- *Signs and Symptoms:*
  - It acts as acid corrosive poisons.
  - There is intense thirst, vomiting and lips are stained brown.
  - Vomiting matter-dark yellow or blue in colour with peculiar odour of iodine.
  - Urine–scanty, red-brown in colour.
- *Fatal dose:* 2-4 gm (30-60 ml of tincture).
- *Fatal period:* 1 to several days.
- *Treatment*
  - Stomach wash with warm water containing soluble starch and albumin or 5% solution of sodium thiosulphate.
- *Chronic Poisoning (Iodism):*

  (c.f. **Plumbism**—chronic lead poisoning.
  Saturnism—chronic lead poisoning.
  Hydrargyrism—*chronic mercury. poisoning*).
  - The symptoms are pain over the frontal sinus, running of nose, conjunctivitis, bronchial catarrh, salivating nausea, vomiting, purging, emanciation, wasting of breasts, testes etc and acne and erythematous patch of the skin.

AGRICULTURAL POISONING

- Insecticide poisoning is most common form of suicide.

ZINC PHOSPHIDE (RAT POISON OR RODENTICIDE)

- It reacts with acid in the stomach and liberates phosphine.
- The symptoms are vomiting, diarrhoea, cyanosis, respiratory distress, fever and death.
- *Fatal dose*: 5 gm.
- *Fatal period*: 24 hours.
- It has a garlic odour.
- *Treatment*
  - Stomach wash with potassium permanganate.
  - Purgatives.

ORGANOPHOSPHORUS POISONS (IRREVERSIBLE INHIBITOR)

- They are derived from phosphoric acid and form two series of compounds:
  - *Alkyl phosphates**
    (i) HETP (ii) TEPP (TEPP is Highly Toxic) (Toxicity: 50 mg I/M 100 mg oral) (iii) OMPA (iv) **Malathion*** (kills bug).
  - *Aryl phosphates**
    i. Parathion (follidol).
    ii. Diazinon (tik–20).
- Insecticides of vegetable origin→Nicotine, Pyrethrins, Rotenone.

Mechanism of Action

- Organophosphorus insecticides **irreversibly inhibit acetyl cholinesterase** by **phosphorylating** and cause accumulation of acetyl choline at muscarinic and nicotinic synapses.

Toxic Effects

They have three distinct toxic effects:

1. The **muscarinic side effects** are **"DUMBBELS":**
   Diarrhoea
   Urination
   Miosis*—contracted pinpoint pupil (c.f. Endrin-dilation of pupils)
   Bronchorrhea (increased tracheobronchial secretions–**Asthma like symptoms)**
   Bradycardia
   Emesis
   Lacrymation
   Salivation
   - **Porphyrinaemia**, resulting chromolachyorrhoea (shedding of red tears)* due to accumulation of porphyrin in the lacrymal gland.

2. **Nicotinic sign include:** Twitching, Fasciculations, Weakness, Hypertension, Tachycardia, Respiratory rate decreased with respiratory failure.
3. **CNS effects:** Anxiety, restlessness, tremor, convulsion, confusion, weakness and coma.

Intermediate Syndrome: Acute Respiratory Paresis and Muscular Weakeness.

- *Fatal dose*: TEPP 140 mg; OMPA 175 mg; Parathion 175 mg; Malathion and diazinon 1 gm orally.
- *Fatal period*: Half to 4 hours.

  Diagnosis

  – **RBC cholinesterase estimation:** Most sensitive and most rapid test but cumbersome. **Plasma Cholinesterase is more commonly done** because its easy and inexpensive test.
- *Treatment:*
  1. ***Atropine,*** a muscarinic receptor antagonist, should be administered for muscarinic effect up to drying of bronchial and mucous membrane secretions.
  2. **Pralidoxime (2-PAM)**, an oxime that **reactivates cholinesterase***, is indicated for nicotinic symptoms in organophosphorus poisoning.
  3. Gastric lavage and contaminated skin is washed with soap and water.
- *Postmortem appearances:*
  – Blood stained froth is seen at the mouth and nose.
  – The stomach content may **smell of kerosene** (due to **Aromax.*** a solvent present in pesticides).
  – Suicide is very common.

CARBAMATES (REVERSIBLE INHIBITOR)

- Carbamate insecticides include carbaryl, aldicard, baygon, ficam and propoxur.
- Carbamates reversibly inhibits acetyl cholinesterase enzyme.
- Atropine is the antidote.

- **Pralidoxime should not be given** because →Carbamate oxime complex are more potent inhibitor of cholinesterase than carbamate alone.
- Artificial respiration and gastric lavage is given.

ENDRIN—PLANT PENICILLIN

- It is a polycyclic, polychlorinated hydrocarbon.
- It is also called (**plant penicillin**).
- PAM is not used in treatment.
- It causes dilated pupils.

Fluoride

- Used as rodenticide.
- Treatment of choice is calcium.

Aluminium Phosphide (Celphos)

- 3 gms of ALP liberates 1 gm of phosphene on contact with moisture, a systemic poison.
- It inhibits **cytochrome C oxidase** of mitochondria or damage by free radicals causes global hypoxia.
- Organs with the greatest oxygen requirements appear to be especially sensitive to phosphine, including the brain, kidneys, heart and liver. Liver shows centrizonal haemorrhagic* necrosis.
  - Phosphine has a characteristic odor described as "decaying fish"/or garlic.
  - Esophageal Strictures and Fistula seen in survivors.
  - Cardiac dysrhythmias probably secondary to electrolyte imbalances have been described in sub-lethal acute exposures.
  - Transient atrial fibrillation and **sub-endocardial infarction.**
  - **Adrenocortical injury** with elevated serum cortisol levels have been reported.
- Treatment of choice is $MgSO_4$ however no specific antidote is given.
- Activate charcoal and paraffin for adsorption and excretion of PH_3 respectively.

  Gastric Lavage fluid + Silver Nitrate = Black Colour (Thanks to **Phosphine**).

METALLIC POISONS

Arsenic

- Metallic arsenic is not poisonous, as it is not absorbed from the alimentary canal.

Poisonous Compounds

1. *Arsenious oxide or Arsenic trioxide (**Sankhya or Somalkar**):* It is known as white arsenic. It has been found to be useful in **treatment** of **Acute Promylocytic Leukemia (APL)*** by inducing an apoptosis also known as programmed cell death.
2. *Copper acetoarsenate (paris green):* It combines with sulphydryl enzymes and interferes with cell metabolism.
3. *Copper arsenate (Schcele's green).*

Signs and Symptoms

1. *The Fulminant type:* Large doses of arsenic can cause death in one to 3 hours from shock.
2. *The Gastroenteric type*: This is acute poisoning, resembling bacterial food poisoning or cholera. **[N.B.: Arsenic can cause Acute Yellow Fatty Liver].**
   - This is the most common form.
   - The stools are expelled frequently and involuntarily, are dark coloured, stinking and bloody, but later becomes colorless, odourless and water resembling **rice water stools of cholera.****
   - Sequence of symptoms:
     – Throat pain.
     – Vomitting (Bile, Blood and Mucous).
     – Purging (Tenesmus present).
3. *Narcotic form:* Tenderness of the muscle, delirium, coma and death.
   - Arsenic poisoning resembles
     – Premalignant condition
     – Cholera

– Fading measles
– Addison's disease.

Killing Style: It's a **Protoplasmic poison** and combines with sulfhydryl groups on enzymes causing disruption. Trivalent arsenic >> toxic Pentavalent Arsenic.

- *Fatal dose:* 0.1 to 0.2 gm or **100 to 200 mg**[AIIMS].
- *Fatal period:* 1-2 days.
- *Treatment*
  1. Freshly prepared precipitated hydrated **ferric oxide** (arsenic antidote)* is given. Dialysed iron is substitute.
  2. In arsenic poisoning **BAL** is an antidote (BAL is contraindicated in **cadmium** and **iron poisoning**).
  3. Calcium disodium versenate.
  4. Alkali is contraindicated.
- *Postmortem appearance*
  – **Red Velvety*** appearance of the stomach mucosa.
  – **Subendocardial haemorrhage** of heart.*
- *Chronic poisoning*
  1. **CNS**—Sensory + Motor (mixed) Polyneuritic, Polyneuritic, optic neuritis. Neuropathy mimicking Guillain-Barré syndrome. **Symmetrical Sensory Neuropathy** with a glove and stocking anaesthesia is diagnostic. **NEET**
  2. **Skin**—Finely mottled brown change mostly on the temples, eyelids and neck **(Rain Drop Pigmentation)**.
     – There may be a rash resembling **fading measles rash***, *(c.f. Barbiturate Blisters, Co Blisters, Meprobamate Blisters).*
     – **Hyperkeratosis and hyperpigmentation** of the palms and soles with irregular thickening of the nails is seen.
     – Nails show ALDRICH MEE's line (Leukoparonychia).{*Confuzer** **Beau's Lines**

→ Chronic Systemic Disease, also **Muehrcke's Line**→ hypo proteinemia}.
– Nails show ALDRICH MEE's line (Leukoparonychia).

Golden Hair seen in Arsenic and Cadmium

- *Arsenophagists* are people who take arsenic daily as tonic or as an aphrodisiac and they acquire a tolerance of up to 0.3gm or more in one dose.

Medicolegal Importance

- Arsenic is the most popular homicidal poison. Also known As (AKA) inheritance powder.
  – Arsenic trioxide (As_2O_3) has been described in the treatment of **acute myeloid leukemia,** AML.
- It delays **putrefaction and cadaveric rigidity.**
- It can be detected in completely decomposed body.
- It can be found in bones, hair and nails for a long time.
- It can be detected in charred bone and ashes.
- **Arsenic doesn't cross BBB (Blood Brain Barrier).**
- It is sometimes used in **abortion sticks.**
- Arsenic causes **Black foot disease***NEET (*cf.* **the pigmentation of skin is brown).**
- Marsh test and Reinsch test are important chemical tests*.
  Early stages greatest quantity in liver (Acute Yellow Fatty Liver).
  Later keratin tissues: BONE, HAIR and NAILS.

Test for Arsenic

I. Reinsch Test–Obsolete.
II. **Marsh Test (mARS**enich**)**–This single test that dethroned Arsenic from being "King of Poisons"–Obsolete.
III. Gutzeit Test.
IV. Neutron activation analysis.
V. Atomic absorption spectroscopy.

MERCURY

- Most poisonous salt of Hg **is mercuric chloride (corrosive sublimate)**.
  - *Symptoms:* Acid metallic taste, hoarse voice, greyish white coating of tongue, blood-stained stool, circulatory collapse, necrosis of jaw, membranous, colitis, **proximal renal tubular necrosis**.*

Acrodynia*(Acro-Limbs and Dynia-Pain) is seen in mercury poisoning **(Pink's Disease)**. It is pain, swelling and parasthesia of limbs.

Mimimata disease—Contamination of fish with mercury, at a place called **Minimate Bay** in Japan.

- *Fatal dose:* 1-4 gm.
- *Fatal period:* 3 to 5 days.
- *Treatment*
  1. Gastric lavage with (sodium formaldehyde sulphoxylate.
  2. BAL (BAL/MER).
  3. Penicillamine (Pencillamines not given in arsenic poisoning).

Chronic Poisoning: (Hydrar Gyrism)

- The symptoms are salivation, sore mouth and throat, fine tremors of the tongue, hands, arms, anemia.
- *Shaking palsy* is associated with Hg poisoning. Mercurial tremors are also called **hatter's shakes or glass blower's shake (Danbury Tremors). Coarse, Intentional Tremors.**
- **Mercurial erethism**** is seen in persons working with mercury in mirror manufacturing firms. Erethism is characterized by shyness, timidity, irritability, loss of confidence, mental depression, loss of memory and insomnia **(Psychological symptoms).**
- *Mercurialentis* is a peculiar eye change due to brownish deposit of mercury through the cornea

on the anterior lens capsule **(Brown-Malt Reflex*).**

- It is bilateral and has no effect on visual acuity.

LEAD (Pb) (PQZ → Metal Poisonous in Native Form)

- *Acute Poisoning:* The symptoms are metallic taste, dry throat, peripheral circulatory collapse, paraesthesias, depression, coma and death.
  - In acute poisoning, lead accumulated in liver.*
- *Fatal dose*: Lead acetate 20 gm; lead carbonate 4 gm.
- *Fatal period:* 1-2 days.
- *Treatment*
  - The combination of BAL and calcium disodium versenare is effective.
- *Chronic poisoning (Plumbism or Saturnism)*
  - Inhalation of lead dust and fumes by makers of white lead, smelters, plumbers, glass-polishers.
  - Chronic poisoning results from a daily intake of one to two mg of lead.
  - The bone marrow is the most sensible target for lead toxicity: The metal interferes with a variety of haeme biosynthetic enzymes, including ALA-D.
- *Signs and Symptoms:*

  A. Anaemia

  In early stage polycythemia and later stage Anaemia (Punctate Basophila).* Anaemia is due to decrease survival of RBCs and inhibition of haeme synthesis.

  B. Basophilic stippling

  - Dark blue spots in cytoplasm of RBCs due to disturbance in porphyrin metabolism.

    Stippled erythrocytes are typical but not specific for lead poisoning, they also appear in:

    - Thalassemia.
    - Vitamin B_{12} deficiency.
    - Pyrimidine 5' nucleotidase deficiency.
    - Toxicity of aniline, arsenic or benzene.

– **Burtonion line:** A stippled blue coloured line present in upper jaw due to lead sulphide* (least toxic compound of Pb[NEET])*.

C. **Colic and constipation (Dry Belly Ache)*:** First described by Hippocrates in 1370 B.C. may mimick the acute abdomen.

D. **Drops, i.e., wrist drop (Radial nerve)** Foot Drop (Deep peronial nerve).
N.B. →Pure Motor Palsy[NEET].

E. **Lead encephalopathy**
- More common in children.
- May present as Status Epilepticus.

F. **Facial pallor**
- Circum oral facial pallar.
- Most consistent and earliest sign of chronic lead poisoning.

Diagnosis

- In poisoning, the concentration of lead in blood is usually between 0.1 to 0.6 mg per 100 ml.
- X-ray evidence of increased radiopaque bands of lines at the metaphyses of long bones is seen in children.
- CPU (Corpoporphyrin in urine), ALAU (Amino-Laevolinic Acid).

Treatment

i. Most effective treatment of plumbism is calcium-disodium versenate.
ii. BAL.
iii. Penicillamine.

COPPER

- **Ptysalism*** is seen in copper poisoning. It is cupious secretion of saliva.
- Chronic copper poisoning resembles **Wilson's Disease** (Hepatolenticular Degeneration).
- **Clapton's Line**→Greenish line seen on the margins of gums due to formation of copper sulphide.

- **Vineyard sprayer's lung:** Occupational disease seen in Vineyard workers due to Bordeaux solution (1-2% copper sulfate solution).

Chronic ophthalmic exposure of Cu results in:

(a) **Chalcosis oculi:** Copper deposition in the cornea, lens, vitreous and retina.
(b) **Kayser-Fleischer ring:** Pigment ring in the peripheral Descemet's membrane.
(c) **Chalcosis lentis:** Greenish lens opacities as anterior **subcapsular cataract** ('sunflower' cataract).
   - *Fatal dose*–15 gm.
   - *Fatal period*–1-3 days.
   - *Treatment:*
     i. Stomach wash with solution potassium ferrrocyanide.*
     ii. N-penicillamine.
     iii. EDTA.
     iv. BAL.

LITHIUM

- In chronic poisoning, concentrations between 3 and 4 m mol/l may be associated with severe toxicity.
- Hemodialysis is indicated for severe intoxication.

ZINC

- **Metal fume fever** or Smelter's fever, Monday morning fever.
- Zinc toxicity resembles with **malarial chills**.*

CADMIUM

- "Itai Itai" Disease–Bone Fractures.
- **PCT Necrosis.**
- **Golden Hair.**
- Bone Pain.

ORGANIC IRRITANT POISONS

Ricinus Communis

- The castor plant *(arandi*)* grows all over India.
- Entire plant is poisonous, containing **toxalbumen ricin**, a water-soluble glycoprotein and a powerful allergen (CBA).
- Ricin is a **biological warfare agent.***
- A toxalbumen or phytotoxin is a toxic protein, which resembles a bacterial toxin in action and causes agglutination of red cells with some hemolysis and is antigenic.

Signs and Symptoms

Symptoms include salivation, bloody diarrhoea, impaired sight, delirium, convulsions, uremia and jaundice.

- *Fatal dose*: 10 seeds; ricin 6 mg.
- *Fatal period:* Two to several days.
- *Treatment:* Gastric lavage, demulcents.

Croton Tiglium *(Jamalghota)*

- Croton tiglium (Jamalghota or **naepala**) seeds contain **crotin**, a toxalbumen, which is not expressed with the oil.

Signs and Symptoms

There is hot burning pain from mouth to stomach, salivation, vomiting, purging, vertigo, prostration, collapse and death.

- *Fatal dose*–**4 seeds; 1.5 cc of oil (20 Drops).**
- *Fatal period:* 6 hours to 3 days.
- *Treatment:* Stomach wash and demulcents.

Abrus Precatorius *(Ratti)*–[*cf. Viper snake*]

- It is also known as **Jeguirity or Indian liquorice (gunchi**[AIIMS 2017] **or ratti).**
- The seeds are egg-shaped, bright scarlet colour with a large **black spot at one end.***
- The seeds contain an active principle **abrin, a toxalbumen,** which is similar to **viperine snake venom** it also contains Abralin, Abric acid.

- All parts of the plant are poisonous.
- Used as a cattle poison by making **Needles (Suis)***.

Signs and Symptoms

- After ingestion, symptoms include abdominal pain, diarrhoea, weakness, cold perspiration, trembling of the hands, weak rapid pulse and rectal bleeding.
- When an extract of seeds is injected under the skin of the animal, inflammation, oedema, oozing of haemorrhagic fluid from the site of puncture, necrosis. The animal drops down after 3 to 4 days.
- *Fatal Dose:* 90 to 120 mg, by injection, 10 gm, orally.
- *Fatal Period:* 3 to 5 days.
- *Treatment:* Injection of anti-abrin. The needle should be dissected out.
- *Poisoning:* The seeds are used for killing cattle, small sharp-pointed spikes or, '**suis**'* are prepared which are then dried in the sun.

ERGOT

- Ergot is the dried sclerotinum of the **fungus Claviceps purpurea,** which grows on cereals like rye, barley, wheat, oats, etc.
- It contains alkaloids, ergotoxin, ergotamine and ergometrine.
- Associated with **St. Anthony's Fire*** (Consumption or **Ryebread** contaminated with Ergot causing burning sensation of limbs.

Signs and Symptoms

- In acute cases, there is nausea, vomiting, diarrhoea, giddiness, tightness in the chest, difficulty in breathing, marked muscular weakness and exhaustion.
- There may be tingling and numbness in the hands and feet, paraesthesias, followed by twitching or cramps in the muscles.

- Bleeding from nose and other mucous surface is common.

Chronic Poisoning (Ergotism)

- There is tingling and numbness of the skin, vasomotor disturbances leading to dry gangrene of the fingers.
- There is a sensation of **insects creeping under the skin** (**tactile hallucination**). This is also known as **Formication.** Formication is seen in:
  - Ergot.
  - Cocaine.
  - Arsenic poisoning.
- *Fatal dose:* One to two gm.
- *Fatal period:* One to several days.
- *Treatment:* Wash the stomach and give purgatives. Vasodilators, e.g., nitrites are useful.

CAPSICUM ANNUM

- Capsicum or chillies (mirch) have a pungent odour and taste and are used as a condiment.
- The active principles are capsaicin and capsicin.
- It acts as an irritant poison.
  - **Hunan's Hand** is seen due to exposure of Capsicin.
- On cut-section of the seeds of capsicum, the embryo appears like **the Figure of '6'.**
- Capsicum seeds resembles **Dhatura.**

SEMECARPUS ANACARDIUM

- **Marking nuts (bhilawa)** are black, heart-shaped with rough projections at the base.
- Their pericap contains an irritant juice which is brownish, oily and acrid but turns black on exposure to air.
- The active principles are semecarpol and bhilawanol.

Signs and Symptoms

- The lesion resembles a **bruise.**

- The juice, when applied externally causes irritation and a painful blister, which contains acrid serum.
- Colour of artificial bruise is **Dark Brown.**
  - *Fatal dose:* 5 to 10 gm.
  - *Fatal period:* 12 to 24 hours.

Calotropis (Snake Charmers' Plant*, Sodom Apple)

Active Principle – Gigantin – Oculotoxic

- The juice is taken by mouth or introduced into uterus on **an abortion stick for criminal abortion** and as a cattle poison.
- Also used as arrow poison. Active principle–Gigantin.
- To produce artificial bruise.
- The juice produces an acrid bitter taste, salivation, dilated pupils, titanic convulsions, collapse and death.
- The **roots of calotropis plant are even poisonous to cobra*.**

Snakes

- The poisonous snakes may be divided into five families:
  1. **Cortalidae**–Pit viper.
  2. **Viperidae (True viper)***–Russel's viper.
  3. **Elapidae**–Cobra and Krait**.
  4. **Hydrophidae**–Sea snakes (All sea snakes are poisonous).
  5. **Colubridae**–Boom stangs, bird snakes.
- In India, **five** are dangerously poisonous to man:
  - King cobra.
  - Cobra.

- Common krait.
- Russell's viper.
- Saw-scaled viper.

- The most **common poisonous snake** is **common krait.**
- **Boa Constrictor** kills by causing Traumatic **Asphyxia.**

Difference between Poisonous and Non-poisonous snakes

S.No.	*Poisonous*	*Non-poisonous*
1. Belly scales	Large and **cover entire breadth**	Small and do not cover entire breadth
2. Head scales	1. Small (vipers) 2. Large and a. If there is an opening between eye and nostril (pit-viper) b. Third labial touches the eye and nasal shields (cobra) c. Central row of scales on back enlarged; under surface of the mouth has only 4 infralabials, the fourth being the largest (kraits)	Head scales large with the exceptions under the poisonous snakes
3. Fangs	Hollow like hypodermic needles	Short and solid
4. Tail	Compressed	Not much compressed
5. Habits	Usually nocturnal	Not so
6. Bite mark	Two long fangs	Several small teeth, two rows of teeth marks*

Snake Venom

1. Ophitoxemia means poisoning by snake venom.
2. Snake Venom (Saliva) ejected from the poison glands (modified parotid glands).
3. Venom of **elapida (cobra, krait) is neurotoxic,** death from respiratory paralysis.

Nature	Snake
1. Neurotoxic	Cobra (Elapidae)
2. Vasculotoxic	Viper (Resemble symptoms of **Abrus***)
3. Musculotoxic	See snake

Clinical Manifestations

The most common manifestation following snake bit (poisonous or non-poisonous) is **fright.**

Cobra

1. Local symptoms start within 6 and 8 minutes.
2. The bitten area is tender with slight burning pain. **Dry bite** is most commonly caused by cobra.
3. The patient feels sleepy, slightly intoxicated, weakness of legs and is unable to stand or move.
4. There may be extra-ocular muscle weakness, ptosis and strabismus.
   Corneal Opacification Syndrome* is seen in cobra snake bite.
   Cobra venom owes its ocular effects to its **cardiotoxin**, the only venom fraction capable of inducing the corneal opacification syndrome.
5. Coma sets in and finally the respiration stops with or without convulsions and the heart stops.

Krait

- There is **no swelling** and burning pain at the site of the bite.

True Viper (Russel Viper)

1. When venom is injected, the spot develops severe pain, the swelling starts within 15 minutes.
2. Tingling and numbness over the tongue and mouth or scalp and paraesthesia around the wound occur.
3. The main feature is **persisting shock.**
4. A haemorrhagic syndrome with blood stained sputum, haemorrhages from gums, rectum, the site of the bite etc. occur due to increased coagulation time.

5. Intravascular haemolysis may lead to **haemo-globinuria** and renal failure.

Sea Snakes

- After half to one hour, the patient develops pain, stiffness, and weakness of the **skeletal** muscles.
- Generalized rhabdomyolysis.

Fatal dose:

- Cobra 12 mg; Russell's viper 15 mg; Echis 8 mg; Krait 6 mg, of dried venom.

Fatal period:

- Cobra half to six hours; viper one to two days.

Treatment

1. Cross-shape incision is given.
2. Bandage should not obstruct arterial or venous circulation.
3. Polyvalent antisnake venom.
   - Dose: 20 ml/IV.
   - Prepared from: Cobra
Russel's viper
Sawscale viper
Common krait
   - Useful only when given within **4 hours.**
   - No use after 24 hours.*

PM Finding

Poisonous snake has 2 or 1 fang marks, non-poisonous semi-circular set.

CANTHARIDES

- **Spanish fly** (blister beetle) is used externally as an irritant, and is commonly popular as an aphro-dosiac.
  - The active principle is **cantharidin.**
  - The Indian fly (beetle) contains about **3% cantharidin**.
  - Cantharidin is readily absorbed from all surfaces including the skin.

- *Fatal dose:* 15 to 50 mg of cantharidin, or 1.5 gm of powdered cantharides.
- *Fatal period:* 24 to 36 hours.

Alcohol

• Absolute Alcohol	99.5%	Alcohol
• Rectified Spirit	90%	Alcohol
• Denatured Alcohol	95%	Alcohol + 5% wood neptha
• 100 Proof ethanol is	50%	Ethanol

Relative Concentration of Alcohol at Equilibrium

• Blood	1 unit
• Urine	1.3 unit
• Alveolar air	.0021 unit
• CSF	1.1 to 1.27

Blood Alcohol Curve

Following consumption of a single alcoholic drink, the combined effects of different factors affecting absorption, metabolism and excretion, result in a characteristic blood alcohol curve:

a. **Absorption Phase:** The alcohol concentration **rises steeply** to a distinct maximum (absorption phase).
   (The peak concentration is reached 45 to 90 minutes after ingestion, the majority after 60 minutes).
b. **Equilibrium Phase:** There then follows an irregularly curved fall due to a period of diffusion within the tissues to equilibrium. This takes place over 15 to 30 minutes.
c. **Elimination Phase:** The BAC then falls progressively in a linear fashion.

The Mellanby Effect*: The behavioural impairment at a given blood alcohol level was greater when the **blood alcohol level was rising** than when it was falling.

Symptomatology

1. **Stage of Excitement**
   - *Alcohol gaze nystagmus*
     - Horizontal Jerking movement in the direction of gaze. Independent of position of heat.
     - Average level of 80 mg% cause alcohol gaze nystagmus.
2. **Stage of Incoordination**
   - It occurs above 150 mg% or 0.15 **(critical level).**
3. **Stage of Coma**
   - **McEvan's sign** is positive: Pupils become constricted but get dilated on pinching/slapping/ painful stimulus.
   - At or above 400 mg% it causes coma.

Stages of Intoxication
1. Excitement (<100 mg%) 2. Confusion (100-200 mg%) 3. Stupor > 200 mg%

Jellinek's Classification of Alcoholism

- **Alpha**→Taking alcohol to relieve pain.
- **Beta**→Heavy drinking.
- **Gamma**→Severe form, withdrawal symptoms are experienced.
- **Delta**→Drinker cannot withstand dry spells (Without alcohol).
- **Epsilon**→Periodically drinking.

Key Points

- **Widmarks equation/formula**

  The Widmark equation gives an approximation of the peak BAC expected following ingestion of a known quantity of alcohol.
  - It was given by Swedish Toxicologist **Eric Prochet Widmark*.**

- It takes into account size, sex and type of alcoholic liquour.
- a = pcr

  r → constant and its value is:

  0.7 → male

  0.65 → female

  p → Body weight

  c → Blood alcohol concentration

  a → Weight of alcohol.

Explanation: According to this equation peak BAC (in mg%) equals alcohol ingested (in grams) × 100, divided by corrected body weight (in kgs × Widmark factor); where the Widmark factor is an estimate of body water content and averages 0.7 for men and 0.65 for women.

Widmark's original research, still valid today, found that the average man's body can hold alcohol in even distribution in 68% of its weight. He called this "0.68" factor as Widmark 'r' factor. The lower-case "r" stands for "reduced body mass", or "reduzierte körpermasse".

Alcohol Withdrawal

Falling BAC after prolonged heavy intake causes cortical and autonomic nervous system excitability.

a. **Uncomplicated alcohol withdrawal**

   Onset follows 6-12 hours after stopping drinking. Peaks at 48 hours. Subsides over next few days.

b. **Alcohol withdrawal fits**

   Onset within 12-24 hours. Generalised fits, of unknown cause.

c. **Alcohol withdrawal delirium (delirium tremens)**

   Severe withdrawal syndrome due to cortical and brainstem hyperexcitability. Onset follows within a week of stopping drinking. Lasts 2-4 days.

Symptoms are typically worse at night. Dehydration and electrolyte disturbances are frequent.

d. **Wernicke's encephalopathy**

An acute, potentially reversible, neurological disorder due to **thiamine deficiency** in alcoholism.

The clinical features include disorientation, clouding of consciousness, ocular abnormalities, nystagmus, ataxia and peripheral neuropathy. Untreated it may be fatal or may progress to chronic Korsakoff psychosis.

e. **Korsakoff psychosis**

A chronic, irreversible psychotic neurological disorder due to the combined effects of alcohol toxicity and metabolic derangement due to thiamine deficiency. May follow Wernicke's encephalopathy. The main clinical features are profound impairment of short term memory, inability to learn new information and compensatory confabulation.

f. **Alcoholic hallucinosis.**

Tests for Estimation of Alcohol

- **Macro Method→*Hine and Kozelka method* (Color/Spot Test).**
- **Micro Method→*Cavett's Test.***
- **Chemical methods**→Based on principle of reduction of **Potassium-bichromate.**
- **Breath analyser test** invented by ***Robert Borkenstein and*** is based on **Henry's Gas law.**

  Level in blood (BAC in milligrams alcohol/100 ml blood) is 2300 times higher than the level in breath (BrAC in micrograms/100 ml breath).

Quick Conversions
BAC = 2.3 × BrAC
BAC = 0.75 × UAC
BAC = VHAC × 0.8
• Blood Alcohol Conc. (BAC)
• Breath AC (BrAC)
• Urine AC (UAC)
• Vitreous Humor AC (VHAC)

(*c.f.* As urine contains a large proportion of water and very little solid material, urine contains more alcohol per 100 ml than does blood.)

- **Gas Chromatography***→Most desirable method for medicolegal purpose.
- **Tryptophan** metabolism is disrupted in chronic alcoholism.
- **Legal Limit** prescribed by Motor Vehicle Act is ***30 mg% of blood alcohol level (BAL).***
- **Critical Limit** leading to in coordination of muscles is ***150 mg% BAL.***
- Rate of fall in BAC is ***15 mg%/hour****, ethyl alcohol follows* ***zero order kinetics.***
- *Sec 510 IPC*→Misconduct due to intoxication.
- Drunkenness is never an excuse, but when drunkenness becomes a disease then it does become a defence, if a crime is committed. For e.g., Delirium Tremens.

Interpretation of Postmortem Blood Alcohol Levels

1. Blood should be taken from peripheral veins **(femoral vein in pelvis)** to avoid possible artifact.
2. Postmortem alcohol production. Activity due to bacteria and yeast present in the blood stream, acting on glucose and lactate, can result in spurious alcohol production in the body (*in vivo*) or within a specimen tube (*in vitro*).

Factors Favouring

- Warm environment.
- Septicaemia (bacteria in bloodstream at time of death).
- Hyperglycaemia (substrate for fermentation), severe disruptive trauma (allows spread of bacteria).

Factors Inhibiting

- Refrigeration.
- Use of Fluoride/Oxalate preservative in collection tube (prevents further fermentation).

Methanol Poisoning

- Methanol may be present in **contaminated country liquor**, used to denature ethanol.
- Metabolized to **formaldehyde and formic acid** by **alcohol and aldehyde dehydrogenase respectively.**
- **It** is a **CNS depressant** and **toxicity** is **mainly due to formic acid.**
- Earliest clinical presentation is **abdominal cramps.**
- It causes **snow-field vision**, blurred vision, decreased visual acuity, diplopia and photopia.
- Severe non-diabetic acidosis in unconscious person is suggestive of methanol poisoning.

  1.25 ml/kg body weight, minimum lethal dose of methanol.

Treatment

- **Haemodialysis** is the treatment of choice.

Antidote

- Ethanol.
- 4-Methyl Pyrazole (Fomipazole) is a specific inhibitor of **Alcohol dehydrogenase**—retards methanol metabolism. Loading dose is 15 mg/kg IV followed by 10 mg/kg every 12 hours till serum methanol falls below 20 g/dl.

  Indication for antidote:

- Methanol conc. >6 mmol/L.
- Increased anion gap acidosis.
- Visual symptoms.

- Folinic acid enhances excretion of formic acid.

Postmortem Findings

- Marked cyanosis.
- Absence of postmortom clotting.
- Haemorrhagic necrosis of putaman is seen.
- **Minimum lethal dose of methanol** is **0.3-1.0 gm/kg.**

Methyl Alcohol Poisoning
Treatment: • **Haemodialysis (treatment of choice).** • $NaHCO_3$ for acidosis and treatment of seizures. • **Ethanol** or **Fomepizole (4-Methyl pyrazole) therapy in:** 1. Methanol conc. >6 mmol/L. 2. Increased anion gap acidosis. 3. Visual symptoms.

Methanol vs. Ethylene Glycol
Methanol: Alcohol dehydrogenase converts into formaldehyde then by aldehyde dehydrogenase to formic acid (Ant's sting). **Ethylene glycol:** Odorless and Sweet. Alcohol dehydrogenase converts **Oxalic Acid**[NEET] (Rust Removers and Ink Remover). Oxalic acid combines with blood calcium to form Envelope or Kidney Shaped–dihydrate crystals of **calcium oxalate** seen in kidneys and urine. Needle-shaped-monohydrate crystals **can damage kidney.**

SOMNIFEROUS POISONS OPIUM

- **Opium (afim*)** is also known as Kasoomba or Madak or Chandu (Poorman's Heroine).
- Opium is the dried juice obtained from the poppy **UnRipe Capsule** (papaver somniferum).

- Opium contains two chemically different groups of alkaloids.
  - The phenanthrenes–morphine 10% **codeine** 0.5% and the baine 0.3%, which are narcotic.
  - The isoquinolines-papaverine 10% and narcotine 6% no narcotic property.
- Thaibine an active principle of opium can cause convulsions.
- The artificial derivatives are heroin, dihydromorphine.
- Opiates exert their effects because of their chemical similarity to natural substances called **endorphins.***
- Opioid drugs are capable of producing physical addiction and also psychological and euphoria.
  - *Fatal dose:* Opium 2 gm; morphine 0.2 g.
  - *Fatal period:* 6-12 hours.

Signs and Symptoms

- **The contact of morphine with the skin of sensitive persons may cause erythema, urticaria and itching dermatitis.**
- It first stimulates, then depresses and finally paralyses the nerve centers.
  - *Stage of excitement:* There is a sense of well being, increased mental activity, freedom from anxiety, talkativeness, restlessness, hallucinations, flushing of face, maniacal condition.
  - *Stage of stupor:* The symptoms are headache, incapacity for exertion a sense of weight in the libs, giddiness, drowsiness and stupor. **Bradycardia is characteristic**[NEET].
  - *Stage of coma:* The patient passes into deep coma from which he cannot be aroused.

The pupils are contracted to pinpoint size and do not react to light, but in late stage they may be found to be dilated.

Treatment:

1. The preferred, more definitive treatment for the typical overdose is the narcotic antagonist naloxone I.V.

2. Stomach wash with a solution of **1 : 500 potassium permanganate (High concentration)**.
3. Atropine is not recommended as it can cause death by paralyzing the motor and sensory nerves like morphine.
4. N-allyl normorphine (lethidrone or nalorphine) is a specific antidote for morphine codeine, pethidine and methadone.
   Nalmephene is one of the latest treatment for opium poisoning.
5. When coma is deep-artificial respiration and oxygen is given.

Postmortem Appearance

- Signs of asphyxia are prominent. Froth is seen at the mouth and nostrils.
- The brain, meninges and abdominal organs are congested.
- Postmortem hypostasis: Black coloured.

Chronic Poisoning (Morphinism; Morphinomania)

- Opium addicts can tolerate 3 to 6 gm per day.
- The habitual use first causes a pleasurable feeling of relief and well being, but as larger doses are taken there is disinterest and recurring periods of depression follow.
- Loss of memory, mental fatigue, gradual intellectual, and moral deterioration occur.

Withdrawal symptoms of opioids tend to be **opposite** to the acute effects of the drug.

- **Yawning**, insomnia, dysphoric mood.
- Dehydration (**Tears, Sweat, Loose Motions, Vomiting, Running Nose).**
- **Increased** BP, Pulse, Resp. Rate, Temperature.
- Pupillary dilation (Mydriasis), **Piloerection**
  [Drug of Choice 1. **Methadone**
  Drug of Choice 2. **Clonidine].**

Chemical Test to Detect the Presence of Opium

- *Marquis test**.
- *Deniges' test.*
- *Husemann's test.*

HEROIN (DIACETYL MORPHINE)

- Also known as: Smack, brown sugar, junk, dope.
- It is white in color.
- **"Cutting In":** Term used for adulteration of heroin.
- Substances used for adulterations:
  - Quinidine
  - Mannitol
  - Fructose
  - Talc
  - Chalk powder.
- Heroin + cocaine is called **"Speed Balls".**

DELIRIANT POISONS (DHATURA, BALLADONNA, CANNABIS)

Datura Fastuosa

- *There are two varieties:*
  - Datura alba–white flowered plant.
  - Datura niger–a deep purple flowered plant.
- The fruits are spherical and have sharp spines (thorn-apple).
- Datura stramonium is known as **thorn apple**.*
- They contain 0.2 to 1.4 of hyoscine (scopolamine), hyoscyamine and atropine.
- **Scopalamine** is one of the active ingredient of **Truth serum** used for **Narco-analysis.**

Signs and Symptoms

All the important signs and symptoms and datura starts with letter 'D'.

1. Dysphagia.
2. Dry and hot skin (hyperpyrexia 103°F body temperature).

3. Diplopia.
4. Dilated pupils (Earliest* feature).
5. Dilated blood vessels resulitng in flushing of face.
6. Delirium:
   - **Muttering delirium*** is present. Irrelevant taking.
   - Pill rolling movement (also seen in parkinsonism).
   - **Carphologia***—picking up of imaginary threads from clothes, bed sheets.
7. Drunken gait.
8. Drowsiness.
9. Death due to respiratory failure.
   - *Fatal dose*: 1gm (100-125 seeds).
   - *Fatal period*: 24 hours.

Treatment

i. Stomach wash with potassium permagnate and weak solution of tannic acid.
ii. Physostigmine is specific in datura poisoning.
iii. Pilocarpine nitrate.
   - *Poisoning:* Crushed or powdered seeds or an extract is used by criminals for stupefying a victim prior to robbery, rape or kidnapping.
     – Road poison/Railway platform poison.*
   - *Mydriatic test*: The pupil dilates within half an hour, if datura is present.

CANNABIS SATIVA OR INDICA

- It is also known as Indian hemp, hashish or marijuana.
- The principal constituent of resin of marijuana is **Tetrahydro cannabinol.*** It is a CNS stimulant.
- It is used in the following forms:
  – *Bhang:* It is prepared from the dried leaves and fruit shoots (**leaves***).
  – *Majoon:* It is a sweet prepared with bhang.
  – *Ganja:* It is prepared from the **flower tops*** of female plant.
  – *Charas or hashish:* It is the resin exuding for the leaves and stems of the plant.

Signs and Symptoms

Large doses cause:

1. *Inebriation:* The person becomes dreamy or semi-conscious and he has realistic vision, usually of sexual nature, e.g., he sees nude beautiful women dancing before him, playing music. It causes psychological high, raises heart rate, delays psychomotor skills.
2. *Narcosis:* There is giddiness and ataxia, tingling and numbness of the skin, general anaesthesia.
   - *Fatal dose: Charas* 2 gm; *Ganja* 8 gm; *Bhang* 10 gm/kilo body weight.
     - *Charas* is the most potent preparation of cannabis.
   - *Fatal period*: Several days.

Chronic Poisoning

- Used in excess, it causes degeneration of CNS.
- There is loss of appetite, weakness, wasting, tremors, vacant look, red eyes, impotence, mental deterioration.
- Rarely, they become insane, and may suffer from hallucinations and delusions of persecution.
- There may be an impulse to kill.

Run Amok (Slang – Going Postal/Killing Spree)

Summary: Amok originated from the Malay word *meng-**amuk***, which roughly defined means "to make a furious and desperate charge" much like the ancient Norse berserker warriors practised before going into battle.

Run amok is seen in **Chronic Cannabis Consumer**. The syndrome of "Amok" is found in the DSM-IV TR. The individual first kills a person against whom he may have real or imaginary enmity and then kills anyone that comes in his way until homicidal tendency lasts. Then he may commit suicide or surrender himself.

Two forms: Beramok (more common) and **Amok.**

Typical amok reactions are preceded by:

1. A prodromal state of dysphoria and tension experienced in conjunction with interpersonal or situational problems.
2. **Changes in visual perception and threatening illusions causing fear and rage are common**.
3. This may be followed by a ***sudden kinetic discharge*** during which randomly aggressive, destructive and homicidal acts are committed.
4. The 'amok run' **ends with suicide**, or alternatively, the exhausted individual may be overpowered, who then may claim **amnesia** for his actions.

   This was well revealed during **Vietnam War** when several American soldiers started suffering from acute toxic psychosis arising out of heavy abuse.

   Cannabis may lead to **A-motivational syndrome.**
5. **Criminal Responsibility:** The person is **not held responsible** for his acts. **Run Amok** is considered a disorder of mind and not intoxication.

COCAINE (AKA BENZOYLMETHYLECGONINE)

- It is obtained from leaves of Erythroxylum coca.
- It is used as a local anaesthetic, as a vaso constrictor.
- The usual route of intake is snorting and skin popping.
- Cocaine and heroin in combination is known as Speed Balls (c.f.→ knockout drops which is chloralhydrate also known as. Dry Wine[NEET] ***sookhee sharab***).

Signs and Symptoms

i. *Stage of excitement:* There is bitter taste, dryness of mouth, depression and fatigue.
ii. *Stage of depression:* Within an hour, respirations become feeble, failure or vascular collapse.

Cocaine increases Epinephrine/Dopamine → sympathomimetics→**dilates pupil**.

- *Fatal dose:* 1-1.5 gm orally.
- *Fatal period:* Few hours.
  - *Treatment:* Amyl nitrite is antidote and given by inhalation.
  - NASAL SWAB is preserved in cocaine poisoning because it is SNORTED.

Black Pigmentation of Tongue and Teeth

- *Cocaine habit:* The patient may suffer from hallucinations, convulsions, delirium and insanity.

Magnan's symptoms or cocaine bug is characteristic, in which there is feeling as if grains of sand are lying under the skin or some small insects are creeping on the skin **(tactile hallucinations).** This phenomenon is also known as formication.

Abstinence Syndrome: Hallmark of physical dependence.

- Abstinence syndrome is seen in opiates, cocaine, barbiturates, sedative hypnotics, alcohol etc.
- Nalaxone is used to test physical dependence of opiates.
- Tremors and muscle twitching sign of opiate abstinence syndrome.
- LSD and cannabis dependence does not produce any significant AS.

Substance Abuse in India

- Most common substance abuse in India – Tobacco.
- Most common illicit substance abuse in India – Cannabis.
- Most common illicit substance abuse in the world – Cannabis.

National Household Survey of Drug and Alcohol Abuse in India

- Tobacco >> Alcohol >> Cannabis >> Opiates. Cannabis is by far the most widely cultivated, trafficked and abused **illicit drug.**
- Most common Date Rape Drug→Alcohol.

FOOD POISONING

Bacterial Food Poisoning

- In the infection type, organisms belong mainly to:
  - Salmonella.
  - Coli.
  - Streptococcus.
  - Shigella.
- In the toxic type, is due to ingestion of preformed toxin in prepared food.
- Exotoxins, e.g., enterotoxin of staphylococci and the botulinum toxin, produce intoxication.

Botulism

- Botulinum toxin is the most lethal toxin.
- There are no symptoms of gastroenteritis.
- It is caused by neurotoxin, an exotoxin of clostridium botulinum multiplied in the food, e.g., tinned meat, fish, fruits etc.
- The fatal dose for an adult is 0.01 mg.
- The toxin paralyses the nerve ending.

Signs and Symptoms

- The incubation period is 12 to 30 hours.
- There is nausea, vomiting, constipation, ocular paresis, thirst, pharyngeal paralysis, salivation, sometimes aphonia.
- Excessive fatigue, diplopia, marked muscular weakness. The patient is conscious till death, which is preceded by coma or delirium.
- Bulbar palsy and descending paralysis is seen.
- Differential diagnosis of botulism includes:

- Tetanus.
- Epilepsy.
- Acute gastroenteritis.

LATHYRUS SATIVUS (Kesari dhal)

- Consumption exceeding 30% of the total diet for more than 6 months; produces lathyrism.
- The active neurotoxic principle is **B(N)-oxalyl aminoalanine–BOAA.**
- The continuous use of L. sativus produces. Neurolathyrism, characterised by progressive spastic *paraplegia*, sphincters sensation and mental faculties are preserved.
- **Chinese Restaurant Syndrome caused because of MGA** Mono Sodium Glutamate.
- It leads to seizures that's why MGA is known to cause **Shudder Attack.**

ARGEMONE MEXICANA

- The oil contains two alkaloids:
  - Sanguinarine, and
  - Dihydro sanguinarine.
- Causes epidemic dropsy.
- **Hyper secretory glaucoma*** is seen in—epidemic dropsy.
- Convulsions are not seen in epidemic dropsy.

SPINAL POISONS

Strychnos Nux Vomica (Dog Bottoms/Pets/ Dogs or Birds Poison)

- Strychnine (kuchila) is a powerful alkaloid obtained from the seeds of the strychnos nux vomica.
- The seeds contain two principal alkaloids–strychnine 1.5% and brucine 1.55%.
- Strychnine poisoning resembles **Tetanus** poisoning.

- The action is particularly noted in **Anterior Horn Cells***, mechanism of action of strychnine poisoning is–post synaptic block. It causes **Release Excitation** by inhibiting **Glycine***.
- In strychnine poisoning convulsions affect all muscles at a time.
- The mouth is covered with froth, frequently blood stained.
- Opisthotonus–The convulsions are most marked in antigravity muscles, so that the body typically arches in hyper extension.
- Emprosthotonus–Sometimes spasm of abdominal muscle may bend the body forward.
- Pleurosthotonus—Spasm of muscles causing body to bend sideway.

Test Done for Strychnine Poisoning

1. **Wenzell's Test** (Confuser→*Wetzel's Test* is done for CO poisoning).
2. Sonnenschein's Test.

- *Fatal dose:* 30-100 mg; one crushed seed.
- *Fatal period:* 1-2 hours.

Treatment

i. Short acting barbiturates.
ii. Diazepam.
iii. Stomach wash with potassium permanganate.
iv. **Acidification** of urine enhances excretion of strychnine.

Postmortem appearance: In strychnine poisoning brain is required to be preserved.

Postmortem caloricity is seen in strychnine poisoning.

Other Useful Facts

- **Socrates** was poisoned by *Hemlock* (Conium Maculatum).
- **Curare** is a peripheral nerve poison.
- Cause of death due to curare poisoning is *Asphyxia* because of paralysis of muscles.

CARDIAC POISONS

- Cardiac poisons are:
  i. Nicotiana tabacum (most common substance of abuse in India). **Tobacco Amblyopia**[NEET] is marketed by a gradual impairment of vision characterised by visual field defects and hindered central vision.
  ii. Digitalis purpurea (Foxgloves).
  iii. Nerium odurum (White Oleander or Kaner)–[Toxicity due to cardiac glycosides, Oleanderin and Neriine].
  iv. Cerbera Thevetia (Yellow oleander) [Toxicity – Thevetin, Revoside, Peruvoside, Nerfolium].
  v. Cerbera odallam (Pilikirbir) [Toxicity–Cereberin, odollin, thevatin].
  vi. Quinine (Ambylopia* characterstic).
  vii. **Aconite** (Sweet Poison/Meetha Zehar/Monks Hood)—Alternate dilatation and contraction of pupil is seen in aconite poisoning called **HIPPUS***. **Hypo-Tension**, Tingling numbness of mouth, **Hyper-Salivation.** [**Memorizer**→Hipputension* low BP]
  viii. Hydrocyanic acid.

HYDROCYANIC ACID

- It is also called prussic acid or cyanogen.
- Amygdaline is the glucoside of vegetable origin found in cyanides.
  Amygdalin is acted upon by **Emulsin** to produce Hydrocyanic acid.
  Linseed yields free **HCN.**
- More than 5% carboxyhaemoglobin is seen in cyanide poisoning.
- Cyanide inhibits the action of:
  - Cytochrome oxidase.
  - Carbonic anhydrase.
- It kills by creating histotoxic or cytotoxic anoxia.
- HCN is colorless gas with bitter almonds smell.
- Binds mitochondrial cytochrome oxidase→ Metabolic acidosis→High plasma lactates **(Histotoxic Hypoxia).**

Signs and Symptoms

- Massive doses may produce sudden loss of consciousness and prompt death from respiratory arrest.
- Erosion and haemorrhages in oesophagus and stomach.
- People suffering from **Achlorhydria*** may not suffer from toxic effect of oral ingestion of potassium cyanide.
- The mouth is covered with foam which is sometimes blood stained.
- Fatal dose of HCN (50 mg) is less than soluble KCN (300 mg).
- Death occurs from respiratory failure.
- *Fatal period:* 2-10 minutes.

PQZ → Lee-Jones Test is used for **Cyanide Poisoning,** based on **Prussian Blue Reagent.**

Treatment

- **Amyl nitrite is used by inhalation. (Therapeutic Methemoglobin induction).**
- Sodium nitrite is given I.V.
- Sodium thiosulphate in 50% solution I.V. converts cyanide to non-toxic thiocyanates.
- Methylene blue I.V. is given in case of life threatening methemoglobinemia (**Chocolate Cyanosis**).
- Dicobalt acetate.
- **Para-Amino Propiophenone (PAPP).***
- Vitamin B_{12} (Hydroxy Cobalamine).

  P.M. appearance: The blood is brick-red* due to formation of cyanmethemoglobin.

[N.B.→Potassium Ferro Cyanide is non poisonous].

ASPHYXIANTS

Carbon Monoxide

- Upper limit of safety of carbon monoxide in air is 0.01%.
- At 4% concentration, most common symptom is **muscular weakness**.
- 50% CO Hb produces symptoms like *alcoholic intoxication*.

- 50%-60% produces syncope or coma with intermittent convulsions.
  - The maximum capacity of CO for combining with Hb is **25 ml/100 blood.**
  - **Lethal Dose:** Dose which produces 60% of carboxyhaemoglobin in proportion to the total blood haemoglobin.
  - This ratio is called **Balthazard-Nicloux poisoning coefficient.**

Test Done for CO Poisoning*

- **Kunkel's Test** (Tannic Acid Test).
- **Wetzel's Test.**
- **Hoppe-Seyler's Test (10% NaOH).**

P.M. Appearance

- A cherry-red coloration of the skin, mucous membranes, areas of hypostasis.
- Fine froth may be seen at mouth and nose.
- **Bilateral Symmetrical Necrosis** of the *lenticular nuclei and punctiform haemorrhages** *in the white matter of brain.*

HYDROGEN SULPHIDE

- It is found in large quantity in sewer–**sewer gas.**
  - Hydrogen Sulphide (H_2S) was the culprit in **Japanese 'Detergent Suicide' technique.**
- Other constituents of sewer gas are CO_2, CH_4, CO etc.

WAR GASES

i. *Vesicant*: Mustard gas, lewisites.
ii. *Asphyxiant:* Chlorine, phosgene.
iii. *Tear gases:* **Chlor acetophenone** (CAP), ethyloidoacetate (K.S.K.) bromobenzyl cyanide (B.B.C.).
iv. *Nerve gases:* They are compounds related to phosphate esters in action and toxicity.
v. *Sternutators:* Gases which causes nasal irritation, e.g., Diphenylamine chlorarsine (**sickening gas**).*

MCQs

1. **Vaccine and sera are included in "Drugs and Cosmetics Rule 1945" under:**
   A. Schedule C B. Schedule E
   C. Schedule F D. Schedule H
2. **For gastric lavage the length of stomach tube introduced is:**
   A. 30 cm B. 40 cm
   C. 50 cm D. 60 cm
3. **Gastric lavage can be performed in poisoning by:**
   A. Sulphuric acid
   B. Strychnine poisoning
   C. Carbolic acid
   D. Kerosene oil
4. **Animal affected by poisons similar to human beings is:**
   A. Rabbit B. Cat
   C. Frogs D. Guinea pig
5. **Pot. permanganate in gastric lavage is used in the strength of:**
   A. 1 : 500 B. 1 : 5000
   C. 1 : 1000 D. 1 : 10,000
6. **Universal antidote contains:**
   A. Mag. oxide, Charcoal and Pot. permanganate
   B. Mag. oxide, Charcoal and Tannic acid
   C. Charcoal, Pot. permanganate and Tannic acid
   D. Pot. permanganate, Mag. oxide and Tannic acid
7. **Dimercaprol is useful in the treatment of poisoning by:**
   A. Opium B. Cyanide
   C. Lead D. Phosphorus

---

1 C 2 C 3 C 4 B 5 B 6 B 7 C

8. Alkalinisation of urine is indicated in poisoning by:
A. Salicylates
B. Opiates
C. Amphetamines
D. Organophosphates

9. Maximum diaphoretic action can be seen with:
A. Salicylates
B. Alcohol
C. Pilocarpine
D. Paracetamol

10. Narcotic drugs and psychotropic substances act repeals:
A. Poison's Act, 1919
B. Dangerous Drugs Act, 1930
C. Drugs and Cosmetic Act, 1940
D. Drugs Control Act, 1950

11. Wall scrappings can be used as a first aid remedy in poisoning by:
A. Hydrochloric acid
B. Oxalic acid
C. Carbolic acid
D. Salicylic acid

12. Concentration of morphine in standard opium is:
A. 5%
B. 7%
C. 10%
D. 15%

13. Alkaloid of opium showing convulsant action is:
A. Morphine
B. Narcoline
C. Papaverine
D. Thebaine

14. Fatal dose of opium in an adult is about:
A. 0.2 gms
B. 0.5 gms
C. 1 gm
D. 2 gm

15. Specific antidote preferred in opium poisoning is:
A. Nalorphine
B. Lavallorphan
C. Naloxone
D. Atropine

---

8 A 9 C 10 B 11 B 12 C 13 D 14 D 15 C

16. Highly addicting drug among the drugs of addiction is:

A. Bhang B. Charas
C. Heroin D. Amphetamine

17. Most common addicting drug used world-wide is:

A. Marijuana B. Brown sugar
C. Alcohol D. Cocaine

18. Reduction in the blood concentration of alcohol per hour is about:

A. 10 mgs% B. 15 mgs%
C. 25 mgs% D. 30 mgs%

19. Quantity of ethyl alcohol present in industrial methylated spirit:

A. 50% B. 80%
C. 90% D. 95%

20. In a female on consumption of same amount of alcohol, the blood alcohol levels in comparison to male of same body weight will be:

A. 10% less B. Equal
C. 10% more D. 25% more

21. Fatal dose of absolute alcohol is:

A. 50 ml to 100 ml B. 100 ml to 150 ml
C. 150 ml to 200 ml D. 200 ml to 250 ml

22. Mc'Evans sign is diagnostic of poisoning by:

A. Cannabis B. Dhatura
C. Alcohol D. Cocaine

23. Alcohol gaze nystagmus becomes apparent with blood alcohol levels above:

A. 10 mgs% B. 20 mgs%
C. 40 mgs% D. 100 mgs%

24. Mostly alcohol is converted in liver to:

A. Acetaldehyde B. Formaldehyde
C. Acetone D. Ether

---

16 C 17 C 18 B 19 D 20 D 21 C 22 C 23 C 24 B

25. Widmarks formula is used to calculate:
A. Blood alcohol level from breath level
B. Blood alcohol level for urinary levels
C. Alcohol consumed for blood alcohol levels
D. Level of intoxication for blood alcohol levels

26. Prohibitory blood level of alcohol as per "Motor Vehicles Act" is above:
A. 10 mgs% B. 30 mgs%
C. 50 mgs% D. 80 mgs%

27. The nerve affected by pressure in "Saturday Night Paralysis" is:
A. Ulnar nerve B. Radial nerve
C. Median N D. Trigeminal N

28. Urinary levels of alcohol in ratio to blood alcohol level is:
A. 1 : 1.3 B. 1 : 1
C. 1.3 : 1 D. 1.6 : 1

29. "Knock out drops" to render a person helpless in robbery is:
A. Dhatura
B. Methaquolone
C. Chloral hydrate/Dry Wine
D. Barbiturate

30. Common substance used as stupefying agent to facilitate robbing or rape is:
A. Chloral hydrate B. Dhatura
C. Cocaine D. Bhang

31. Muttering delirium is seen in poisoning by:
A. Bhang B. Charas
C. Organophosphates D. Dhatura

32. In dhatura poisoning stomach wash normally should be done with:
A. Pot. permanganate B. Lime water
C. Glycerine D. Tannic acid

33. Antidote preferred in *dhatura* poisoning is:
A. Physostigmine B. Pilocarpine
C. Neostigmine D. Morphine

25 C 26 B 27 B 28 C 29 C 30 B 31 D 32 D 33 A

34. Hot as hare, blind as bat, dry as bone, red as beet and mad as wet hen is seen in poisoning by:

A. Atropa belladonna
B. LSD
C. Cocaine
D. Mescaline

35. Active form of the active principle of *bhang*:

A. Cannabinol
B. Cannabidiol
C. Tetrahydro cannabinol
D. Tetrahydro cannabinolic acid

36. Ganja is a preparation made from cannabis using:

A. Dried leaves
B. Flowering tops of female plant
C. Sweet preparation with leaves
D. Resin from stem and leaves

37. "Run amok" condition may be seen in chronic poisoning by:

A. Dhatura
B. Cocaine
C. Cannabis
D. Opium

38. Magnum's symptoms are seen in chronic poisoning by:

A. Dhatura
B. Cocaine
C. Cannabis
D. Opium

39. Red colored tears may be seen in acute poisoning by:

A. Dhatura
B. Heroin
C. Organophosphorus
D. Cocaine

40. Physical dependence is normally not produced by:

A. LSD
B. Heroin
C. Morphine
D. Cocaine

41. Black coloured teeth may be seen in chronic users of:

A. Charas
B. Cocaine
C. Brown sugar
D. Mescaline

---

34 A 35 C 36 B 37 C 38 B 39 C 40 A 41 B

42. Epidemic dropsy is caused by consuming:
A. Argemone oil
B. Lathyrus sativus
C. Mustard oil
D. Nux vomica

43. Small of bitter almonds is present in poisoning by:
A. Prussic acid
B. Phosphorus
C. Oxalic acid
D. Arsenic

44. Amygdalin is hydrolyzed by emulsion into:
A. T.H. cannabinolic acid
B. Hydrocyanic acid
C. BOAA(B) (N) oxalyl amino-alanin (E)
D. Dihydrosanguinarine

45. Hippus sign may be seen in poisoning by:
A. Cocaine
B. Aconite
C. HCV
D. Heroin

46. Cyanide act in the body by:
A. Combining with SH group of mitochondrial enzymes
B. Inhibiting to cytochrome oxidase
C. Forming cyanmethemoglobine
D. Forming thiocyanate

47. Haemodialysis is used in all poison *except:*
A. Alcohol
B. Barbiturates
C. Aspirin
D. Kerosene

48. Usual fatal period in poisoning by pot. cyanide is:
A. Immediate
B. 1 to 2 mts
C. 2 to 10 mts
D. About 30 mts

49. Affinity of carbon monoxide in comparison with oxygen for haemoglobin is:
A. Half
B. Equal
C. 100 time
D. 200 time

50. Hypostasis is cherry-red in colour, in poisoning with:
A. Carbon monoxide
B. Hydrogen sulphide
C. Aniline
D. Phosphorus

---

42 A 43 A 44 B 45 B 46 B 47 D 48 D 49 D 50 A

51. Blistering gas used during wars is:
A. Mustard gas
B. Phosgene
C. Chloropicrin
D. Chloroacetophenone

52. Dicobalt acetate is drug of choice in the treatment of poisoning by:
A. Lead
B. Mercury
C. Cyanide
D. Aluminium phosphide

53. Methyl alcohol excretion from body is mainly through:
A. Urine B. Breath
C. Bile D. Faeces

54. Greatest danger in sewer gas poisoning is from:
A. Ammonia B. Carbon dioxide
C. Hydrogen sulphide D. Methane

55. Antidote used in mushroom poisoning is:
A. Physostigmine B. Atropine
C. Nalorphine D. Meperidine

56. Most potent preparation of cannabis is:
A. Bhang B. Majun
C. Ganja D. Hashish

57. Road traffic accidents from alcoholic intoxication are mostly due to its effects on:
A. Memory B. Thinking
C. Judgement D. Perception

58. Alcohol initially causes depression of:
A. Conduct and judgement
B. Vital centers
C. Co-ordination
D. Emotions

51 A 52 C 53 B 54 C 55 B 56 D 57 C
58 A

59. Hallucinogenic drugs include following *except:*
A. Mescaline
B. Psylocybin
C. Phencyclidine
D. Methadone

60. The term "Speedballs" in addition is used for combination of:
A. Heroin and strychnine
B. Brown sugar and quinine
C. Heroin and cannabis
D. Brown sugar and cocaine

61. Heroin is also known as following *except:*
A. Smack
B. Junk
C. Dope
D. Speed

62. Brown discolouration of the mucosa of the stomach is seen in poisoning due to:
A. Nitric acid
B. Sulphuric acid
C. Hydrochloric acid
D. Mercury
E. Arsenic

63. Amyl nitrite is used as an antidote in .... poisoning.
A. CO_2
B. CO
C. Cyanide
D. Nitric acid
E. Arsenic

64. Complication of kerosene poisoning:
A. Pneumonia
B. Vomiting
C. Hemoptysis
D. Diarrhoea
E. Acute renal failure

65. What poisoning retards putrefaction?
A. Phosphorus
B. Arsenic
C. Mercury
D. Lead
E. Copper

66. Diwali poisoning is due to:
A. Phosphorus
B. Arsenic
C. Mercury
D. Lead
E. Copper

---

59 D 60 D 61 D 62 A 63 C 64 A 65 B 66 A,C

67. Antidote for sodium nitrate poisoning is:
- **A.** Methylene blue IV
- **B.** Egg albumen
- **C.** EDTA
- **D.** Animal charcoal

68. Nux Vomica is:
- **A.** Vegetable poison containing atropine
- **B.** Seed containing strychnine
- **C.** Used as a cattle poison
- **D.** Used to induce vomiting in poisoning

69. Acrodynia is seen in ..... poisoning.
- **A.** Hg
- **B.** Pb
- **C.** Zn
- **D.** As

70. Pin point pupils is seen in .... poisoning.
- **A.** Barbiturate
- **B.** Morphine
- **C.** Organophosphorus
- **D.** Methyl alcohol

71. Nalorphine is used as an antidote of:
- **A.** Strychnine
- **B.** Opium
- **C.** Datura
- **D.** Cocaine

72. Greenish urine is seen in poisoning with:
- **A.** Carbolic acid
- **B.** Nitric acid
- **C.** Copper sulphate
- **D.** Hydrochloric acid

73. Optic atrophy can be caused by .... poisoning.
- **A.** Phosphorus
- **B.** Ethyl alcohol
- **C.** Methyl alcohol
- **D.** Lead

74. Preservative used for alcohol poisoning is:
- **A.** Formalin
- **B.** Saturated solution of sodium chloride
- **C.** Methyl alcohol
- **D.** None of the above

---

67 A 68 B 69 A 70 B 71 B 72 A 73 C 74 B

75. Blue line on the gums is seen in chronic .... poisoning.

A. Hg B. Pb
C. Ag D. As

76. Anaemia, punctate basophilia, constipation blue line and abdominal colic are characteristics of:

A. Opium addiction
B. Arsenic poisoning
C. Mercuric poisoning
D. Lead poisoning

77. In chronic alcoholism which of the following is seen?

A. Delirium tremens
B. Wernicke's syndrome
C. Korsorkoff psychosis
D. All of the above

78. Dilated pupil, dry mouth is a feature of poisoning due to:

A. Morphine
B. Organophosphorous
C. Dhatura
D. Phenothiazines

79. The pupil is constricted in:

A. Dhatura B. Opium
C. Benzodiazepines D. Phenothiazines

80. Best method of treatment of methyl alcohol poisoning is:

A. Calcium gluconate
B. Ethyl alcohol
C. Amphetamines
D. 4-Methy pyrazone

81. The non-poisonous salt of cyanide is:

A. Potassium cyanide
B. Sodium cyanide
C. Hydrocyanic acid
D. Potassium ferrocyanide

75 B 76 D 77 D 78 C 79 B 80 D 81 D

82. **Tactile hallucinations is seen in chronic poisoning with:**
A. Cocaine B. Opium
C. LSD D. Cannabis

83. **Anterior horn cells are affected in:**
A. Datura poisoning
B. Strychnine poisoning
C. Botulism
D. None of the above

84. **An overdosage of morphine is treated with:**
A. Nalorphine IV
B. Steroids
C. IV methadone
D. Naloxone IV

85. **Which of the following toxins can be detected in burnt bone?**
A. Cyanide B. Arsenic
C. Mercury D. Phosphorus

86. **Hatter's Shake is seen in .... poisoning.**
A. Arsenic B. Mercury
C. Phosphorus D. Lead

87. **The non-poisonous salt of cyanide is:**
A. Potassium cyanide
B. Hydrocyanic acid
C. Sodium cyanide
D. Potassium ferro cyanide

88. **Which of the following is a non-poisonous snake?**
A. Viper B. Krait
C. Sea snake D. Rat snake

89. **True about strychnine poisoning is:**
A. All muscles affected at the same time
B. Shoulder girdle affected first
C. Pelvic girdle affected first
D. None of the above

---

82 A 83 B 84 D 85 B 86 B 87 D 88 D 89 A

90. Critical level of alcohol on blood should be:
A. 0.1% B. 0.15%
C. 0.2% D. 0.3%

91. People suffering from achlorhydria may not suffer from toxic effects of oral ingestion of:
A. Phosphorus
B. Copper sulphate
C. Arsenic trioxide
D. Potassium cyanide

92. Shaking palsy is associated with poisoning with:
A. Lead B. Mercury
C. Arsenic D. Strontium

93. Poisoning by irritants may be mistaken for:
A. Peritonitis
B. Cholera
C. Gastroenteritis
D. Intestinal obstruction

94. Antidote for acute iron poisoning:
A. Desferoxamine
B. Na EDTA
C. BAL
D. Penicillamine

95. The following are true about chloral hydrate *except:*
A. Peculiar pungent odour
B. Crystalline
C. Used as hypnotic
D. Sweetish taste

96. At the following blood carbon monoxide concentration the clinical picture will simulate alcoholic intoxication:
A. 10% B. 70%
C. 30% D. 50%

90 B 91 D 92 B 93 C 94 A 95 D 96 D

97. Minimum quantity of blood required to be preserved for chemical analysis is:

A. 2 ml B. 10 ml
C. 50 ml D. 100 ml

98. A pinch of which of the following poisons can kill as many as five persons?

A. Arsenic trioxide
B. Copper sulphate
C. Lead sulphate
D. Arsenic disulphide

99. Which of the following is used in forgeries as an ink remover solution?

A. Sulphuric acid
B. Nitric acid
C. Carbolic acid
D. Oxalic acid

100. It is true about formalin:

A. That it can be used as preservative in alcohol poisoning
B. Never used as a preservative for chemical analysis
C. Used as a preservative in poisoning with digitalis
D. None of the above

101. Which of the following is known as 'Thorn apple'?

A. Dhatura alba
B. Dhatura niger
C. Dhatura stramonium
D. Dhatura metet

102. In Nux Vomica poisoning the following is also required to be preserved:

A. Long bones
B. Brain
C. Muscles
D. Skin

---

97 B 98 A 99 D 100 B 101 C
102 B

103. The following is also known as "knock out drops" or "Micky Finn":

A. Chloroform B. Methyl alcohol
C. Chloral hydrate D. Ethylene glycol

104. *Ganja* is obtained from:

A. Dried leaves B. Fresh leaves
C. Flowering tops D. Roots

105. In carbamate poisoning all the following should be administered *except:*

A. Atropine
B. Artificial respiration
C. Gastric lavage
D. Oximes

106. Fatal period in sulphuric acid poisoning is:

A. 2-4 hours B. 6-10 hours
C. 12-16 hours D. 18-24 hours

107. Blood cholinesterase level should be estimated for three weeks, in non-fatal cases of poisoning with:

A. Parathion
B. Endrine
C. Thallium sulphate
D. Arsenious oxide

108. Atropine should never be started when the patient is cyanosed due to the danger of:

A. Cerebral edema
B. Respiratory arrest
C. Ventricular fibrillation
D. None of the above

109. C.S.F. is required to be preserved in:

A. Alcohol poisoning
B. Arsenic poisoning
C. Copper poisoning
D. Organophosphorous poisoning

---

103 C 104 C 105 D 106 D 107 A
108 C 109 A

110. Large bones of about 6 inches are required to be preserved in:
- **A.** Arsenic and antimony poisoning
- **B.** Aconite poisoning
- **C.** Datura poisoning
- **D.** Smack poisoning

111. An addict develops delusions, misleading hallucinations of sight and hearing and the feeling of creeping things of "grains of sand" in the skin, he is addicted to:
- **A.** Heroin
- **B.** Methaqualone
- **C.** Cocaine
- **D.** Amphetamines

112. About 20 grams of hair are required to be preserved in:
- **A.** Minerals poisoning
- **B.** Aconite poisoning
- **C.** Iodine poisoning
- **D.** Codeine poisoning

113. Which of the following is not used in methyl alcohol poisoning?
- **A.** Gastric lavage
- **B.** Dialysis
- **C.** Ethyl alcohol
- **D.** High dose of vitamin B_{12}

114. In salicylate poisoning the treatment recommended is:
- **A.** Forced diuresis
- **B.** Chelating agents
- **C.** Atropine
- **D.** Conservative

115. Average fatal dose of croton oil seeds is:
- **A.** 500 seeds
- **B.** Handful of seeds
- **C.** About 4 to 5 seeds
- **D.** 20 seeds

---

110 A 111 C 112 A 113 A,D
114 A 115 C

116. Amyl nitrite is an antidote for poisoning with:

A. $H_2 SO_4$
B. Ammonia
C. HCN
D. Carbon monoxide

117. In burnt bones, the following can be detected:

A. Arsenic
B. Lead
C. Organophosphorus compound
D. None of the above

118. The cause of death in cyanide poisoning is:

A. Anoxic anoxia
B. Anaemic anoxia
C. Histotoxic anoxia
D. Stagnant anoxia

119. Which of the following is considered as an antidote for cocaine poisoning?

A. Phenobarbitone
B. Morphine
C. Amyl nitrate
D. Ether

120. Which of the following is considered as an "ideal infanticidal poison"?

A. Cannabis
B. Cocaine
C. Opium
D. Alcohol

121. Teeth are chalky white and brittle in poisoning by:

A. Sulphuric acid
B. Nitric acid
C. Hydrochloric acid
D. Carbolic acid

---

116 C 117 A 118 C 119 C 120 C
121 A

122. Nux vomica seeds contain 2 alkaloids, strychine and ....

A. Hyosine B. Hyocyamine
C. Brucine D. Atropine

123. In low concentration of carbon monoxide (4%), the most common symptom is:

A. Nausea B. Headache
C. Muscular weakness D. Ringing in ears

124. Lungs are preserved in:

A. Alcohol poisoning
B. HCN poisoning
C. Carbon monoxide poisoning
D. All of the above

125. The following alkaloids are present in opium, *except:*

A. Hyoscyamine B. Morphine
C. Papaverine D. Narcotine

126. The treatment of choice in dicoumarol poisoning is:

A. Heparin
B. Aminocaproic acid
C. Vitamin K
D. Vitamin C

127. Chromolacryorrhoea (shedding of pink tears due to accumulation of porphyrin) may be seen in poisoning with:

A. Arsenic
B. Barbiturate
C. $CuSO_4$
D. Organophosphorus

128. Which of the following is the lateral curve of the body in strychnine poisoning?

A. Opisthotonus
B. Emprosthotonus
C. Pleurosthotonus
D. None of the above

---

122 C 123 C 124 D 125 A 126 C
127 D 128 C

129. Which of the following is also known as 'Kasoomba', or 'Madak', or 'Chandu'?

A. Dhatura B. Cannabis
C. Opium D. Calotropis

130. Magnan's symptom is:

A. Illusion
B. Delusion
C. Formication
D. Depersonalisation

131. Which of the following is considered as an antidote for cocaine poisoning?

A. Oxygen B. Diazepam
C. Ethyl alcohol D. Nitric oxide

132. The fatal dose of absolute alcohol in an adult is:

A. 30 ml B. 60 ml
C. 90 ml D. 150 ml

133. The treatment of choice in dicoumarol poisoning is:

A. Aminocaproic acid
B. Heparin
C. Vitamin K
D. Vitamin C

134. The alcohol content in 'Absolute alcohol' is:

A. 90% B. 95%
C. 99.95% D. 100%

135. The active principles of dhatura are all of the following *except:*

A. Pyrocatachol B. Hyocyamine
C. Atropine D. Hyoscine

136. The average fatal period of copper poisoning is:

A. 30-60 minutes B. 1-3 days
C. 3-7 days D. 7-14 days

---

129 C 130 C 131 B 132 D 133 C
134 C 135 A 136 B

137. **While despatching blood and urine for chemical analysis sodium flouride is added as preservative in the following concentration:**
A. 30 mg/10 ml
B. 40 mg/10 ml
C. 50 mg/10 ml
D. 100 mg/10 ml

138. **Ptysalism is seen in:**
A. Arsenic poisoning
B. Copper poisoning
C. Dhatura poisoning
D. Atropine sulphate

139. **The most common death by suicide is by:**
A. Phenobarbitone
B. Insecticide
C. Hanging
D. Suicidal cut throat

140. **Which of the following tests are used for arsenic poisoning?**
A. Marsh's test
B. Reinsh's test
C. Macewen's test
D. Marqui's test
E. Foder's test

141. **Widmark's formula is used to calculate the quantity of the following in the body after equilibrium between the blood and tissues is reached:**
A. Methyl alcohol
B. Nitrous oxide
C. Ethyl alcohol
D. Lithium carbonate

142. **The fatal period of aconite is usually:**
A. 5-10 minutes B. 15-30 minutes
C. 1-5 hours D. 24-48 hours

137 C 138 B 139 B 140 A,B
141 C 142 C

143. All of the following are aryl phosphates *except:*
- **A.** Folidol
- **B.** Parathion
- **C.** Diazionon (Tick 20)
- **D.** Malathion

144. Arsenophagists are:
- **A.** Criminals using arsenic for homicidal purposes
- **B.** Persons using arsenic as abortion stick
- **C.** Person who can tolerate high doses of arsenic after taking arsenic in low doses at frequent intervals
- **D.** Persons using it as cattle poison

145. The upper limit of safety for carbonmonoxide in air is:
- **A.** 0.2%
- **B.** 0.01%
- **C.** 0.4%
- **D.** 0.005%

146. Narcotic drugs and psychotropic substances act was passed in the year:
- **A.** 1981
- **B.** 1983
- **C.** 1985
- **D.** 1986

147. Velvety appearance of stomach is seen in poisoning with:
- **A.** Abrus precatorius
- **B.** Barbiturate
- **C.** Arsenic
- **D.** Lead

148. All of the following causes constriction of pupil *except:*
- **A.** Datura
- **B.** Morphine
- **C.** Organophosphorous poisoning
- **D.** Pontine haemorrhage

149. Following drug causes delirium:
- **A.** Dhatura
- **B.** Cannabis
- **C.** Morphine
- **D.** Barbiturates

---

143 D 144 C 145 B 146 C 147 C
148 A 149 A

150. Macewan's sign is associated with:

A. Alcohol poisoning
B. Pontine haemorrhage
C. Cerebellar tumours
D. Cocaine intoxication

151. Leading questions are permitted only in:

A. Examination in chief
B. Cross examination
C. Dying declaration
D. Re-examination

152. Morphine withdrawal is characterized by all *except:*

A. Miosis
B. Muscle aches and body pain
C. Yawning
D. Rhinorrhea

153. Antidote for oxalic acid poisoning:

A. BAL
B. Animal charcoal
C. Calcium gluconate
D. Magnesium sulphate

154. Which metal poisoning can be detected by analysing bone?

A. Arsenic B. Nickel
C. Chromium D. Lead
E. Mercury

155. Fatal dose of methanol:

A. 15 ml B. 30-60 ml
C. 60-250 ml D. 500 ml

156. What is not seen with bite of pit viper?

A. CVS collapse
B. Absence of local signs
C. Convulsions
D. None of the above

---

150 A 151 B 152 A 153 C 154 A
155 B 156 C

157. Hyperpigmentation of palms and soles is seen in which poisoning?
A. Arsenic B. Mercury
C. Lead D. Copper

158. Carbolic acid poisoning; postmortem findings are:
A. Greenish stomach
B. Yellow charred stomach
C. Leathery stomach
D. Black charred stomach

159. Marsh test used in diagnosis of poisoning due to:
A. Arsenic B. Lead
C. Iron D. Copper sulphate

160. Haemoglobinuria is seen in all *except:*
A. Copper sulphate poisoning
B. Snake venom
C. Clostridium welchii sepsis
D. Thalassemia

161. Marsh test is used for detection of:
A. Arsenic B. Lead
C. Strychnine D. Opium

162. Opium poisoning produces ..... type of respiration.
A. Rapid and shallow
B. Rapid and deep
C. Shallow
D. Diaphragmatic

163. Arsenic poisoning mimics:
A. Cholera B. Food poisoning
C. Alcohol withdrawl D. Tetanus

164. 'Liquid gold' with reference to urine is presence of:
A. Cocaine B. Amphetamine
C. Heavy metals D. Phosphorus

---

157 A 158 C 159 A 160 D 161 D
162 C 163 A 164 B

165. Postmortem cherry red discoloration is due to:

A. Asphyxia
B. Carbon monoxide poisoning
C. Drowning
D. Organophosphorus poisoning

166. Run amok (Homicide delusion) is characteristic of:

A. Cannabis
B. Cocaine
C. Dhatura
D. Alcohol poisoning

167. Almond like bitter smell is positive in:

A. Chloral hydrate poisoning
B. Hydrocyanic acid
C. Hyocymus poisoning
D. Oleander poisoning

168. Dryness of mouth, dilated pupil and delirium are symptoms of:

A. Chronic lead poisoning
B. Opium addiction
C. Chronic arsenic poisoning
D. Dhatura poisoning

169. Heavy metal poisoning cause proximal tubular necrosis:

A. Hg B. Cadmium
C. Lead D. Gold

170. Erethism is seen in which poisoning?

A. Mercury B. Arsenic
C. Aconite D. Phenol

171. Proximal convoluted tubule necrosis is seen in .... poisoning.

A. Phenol B. Arsenic
C. Aconite D. Lead

165 B 166 A 167 B 168 D 169 A
170 A 171 A

172. Paris green is a:
A. Stomach poison B. Contact poison
C. Repellent D. Rodenticide

173. Almond bitter smell is seen with:
A. Cyanide poisoning
B. Arsenic poisoning
C. Lead poisoning
D. None of the above

174. Sodium fluoride is used for preservation of which poisoning?
A. Strychnine B. Oxalic acid
C. Alcohol D. Carbolic acid

175. Haemodialysis is done in all *except* .... poisoning.
A. Barbiturates B. Salicylates
C. Kerosene D. Alcohol

176. In acute organophosphorus poisoning, which of the following is seen?
A. Dry lungs
B. Edematous lungs
C. Pneumonia
D. Pleural rub

177. Widmark formula is used for which poisoning?
A. Alcohol B. Mercury
C. Cyanide D. Lead

178. Asthma like symptoms is seen in .... poisoning.
A. Arsenic
B. Organophosphorus
C. Lead
D. Gold

179. Gastric lavage is contraindicated in .... poisoning.
A. Kerosene B. Carbolic acid
C. Alcohol D. Salicylate

---

172 A 173 A 174 C 175 C 176 B
177 A 178 B 179 A

180. Average fatal period of copper poisoning:
A. 4 hours B. 18-36 hours
C. 24-48 hours D. > 5 days

181. In barbiturate poisoning which is not present?
A. Hypotension
B. Hypothermia
C. Pupils not reactive
D. Pulmonary edema
E. None of the above

182. Morbid jealousy is diagnostic of:
A. Cocaine
B. Cannabis
C. Alcoholism
D. Tobacco intoxication
E. Barbiturate

183. Acute lead poisoning in child presents as:
A. Status epilepticus
B. Ataxia
C. Focal deficit
D. Papilloedema

184. Erethism is seen in toxicity of:
A. Arsenic B. Mercury
C. Lead D. Iron

185. Putrefaction is retarded by:
A. Carbolic acid
B. Oxalic acid
C. Organophosphorous poison
D. Hydrochloric acid

186. Venom of sea snake is mostly:
A. Neurotoxic B. Haemolytic
C. Myotoxic D. Hepatotoxic

187. Widmark formula is used for:
A. Alcohol B. Barbiturate
C. Cannabis D. Opium

---

180 B 181 C 182 C 183 A 184 A
185 A 186 C 187 A

188. Rectified spirit not used as preservative in case of:

A. Phenol
B. Cyanide
C. Insectides
D. Aluminium phosphide

189. Perforation of stomach is more common due to ingestion of:

A. Nitric acid
B. Sulphuric acid
C. Hydrochloric acid
D. Carbolic acid

190. Metal fume fever is common in chronic poisoning with:

A. Mercury
B. Lead
C. Zinc
D. Thallium

191. Least toxic compound of lead is:

A. Lead arsenate
B. Lead oxide
C. Lead carbonate
D. Lead sulphide

192. All of the following are used during heroin withdrawal *except:*

A. Disulfiram
B. Methadone
C. Clonidine
D. None of the above

193. Linseeds used for (cattle/animal) poisoning contain which of the following principle poisoning substance?

A. Aconitine
B. Hydrocyanic acid
C. Pilocarpine
D. Atropine

194. Narcotic abuse case with jet black tongue, the cause is:

A. Cocaine poisoning
B. Morphine poisoning
C. Cannabis toxicity
D. LSD poisoning

---

188 A 189 B 190 C 191 D 192 A
193 B 194 A

195. Patient is brought to casualty with poisoning. Stomach wash lavage fluid on heating produced black precipitate. The poison is:

A. TIC 20 B. $AgNO_3$
C. Malathione D. Cellophose

196. Most specific test for organophosphorous poisoning is:

A. RBC cholinesterase level
B. Plasma cholinesterase level
C. RBC uroporphyrin level
D. Measurement of serum levels of organophosphorous

197. Alternate contraction and dilatation of pupil is seen in .... poisoning.

A. Aconite
B. Cyanide
C. Hemlock
D. Organophosphate

198. Non irritant gas with systemic toxicity:

A. N_2 B. CO
C. NH_3 D. C_2
E. HCl

199. In acute arsenic poisoning, arsenic concentrates in:

A. Liver B. Kidney
C. CNS D. Keratin tissue

200. Hematuria is caused by the bite of:

A. Rusell's viper B. Krait
C. Cobra D. Sea snake

201. In mercury poisoning all are true, *except*:

A. 0.5 g is invariably fatal
B. Death is due to cardiac toxicity
C. Cutaneous reaction can occur
D. None of the above

---

195 B 196 A 197 A 198 B 199 A,B,D
200 A 201 A

202. In a suspected case of death due to poisoning where cadaveric rigidity is lasting longer than usual, it may be a case of poisoning due to:

A. Lead
B. Arsenic
C. Mercury
D. Copper

203. Cyanide poisoning acts by:

A. Inhibiting DNA synthesis
B. Inhibiting enzymes of protein synthesis
C. Inhibiting cellular respiration
D. Inhibiting protein breakdown

204. "Sankhya" used as homicidal poison is:

A. Copper sulphate
B. Aluminum phosphide
C. Arsenious oxide
D. Mercuric chloride

205. Antidote used while doing gastric lavage in acute arsenic poisoning is:

A. Pot. permanganate
B. Hydrated ferric oxide
C. Pot. ferrocyanide
D. Ferrous sulphate

206. Poison which can be detected in burnt bones is:

A. Lead
B. Arsenic
C. Copper
D. Mercury

207. Red salt of arsenic is:

A. Arsenic bisulphide
B. Arsenic trisulphide
C. Copper arsenite
D. Arsenic trioxide

208. In acute arsenic poisoning, maximum concentration of arsenic is detected in:

A. Muscles
B. Liver
C. Kidneys
D. Keratin tissues

---

202 B 203 C 204 C 205 B 206 B
207 A 208 B

209. Route of administration of BAL is:
A. Inhalation B. Oral
C. Intramuscular D. Intravenous

210. Mee's lines are seen in:
A. Teeth B. Nails
C. Bones D. Cornea

211. Milk rose complexion followed by hyper-pigmentation is seen in chronic poisoning by:
A. Mercury B. Arsenic
C. Copper D. Iron

212. Ulcerative gingivitis and necrosis of mucous membrane is seen in poisoning by:
A. Mercury B. Arsenic
C. Copper D. Lead

213. Hatter's shake is seen in chronic poisoning by:
A. Arsenic B. Copper
C. Lead D. Mercury

214. Malt-Brown reflex in chronic mercury poisoning by slit-lamp examination is demonstrable from:
A. Ant. surface of cornea
B. Post. surface of cornea
C. Ant. lens capsule
D. Post. lens capsule

215. Chemical antidote used in acute mercury poisoning is:
A. Sod. formaldehyde sulphoxylate
B. Ferric oxide
C. Pot. ferrocyanide
D. Mag. sulphate

216. Excretion of poison by colonic mucous membrane is in poisoning by:
A. Arsenic B. Lead
C. Mercury D. Copper

209 C 210 B 211 B 212 A 213 D
214 C 215 A 216 C

217. Feature most commonly encountered in chronic lead poisoning is:
A. Lead line B. Lead palsy
C. Dry belly aches D. Encephalopathy

218. Burtonian line is seen in the chronic poisoning by:
A. Arsenic B. Copper
C. Mercury D. Lead

219. 'Sindhur' used by ladies is:
A. Lead acetate B. Lead tetraoxide
B. Lead chromate D. Lead carbonate

220. Anaemia, with punctate basophilia is seen in chronic poisoning by:
A. Lead B. Copper
C. Iron D. Arsenic

221. In chronic lead poisoning, diagnostic increase in urinary levels are of:
A. Corpoporphyrin B. Urobilinogen
C. Bile D. Calcium

222. Usual fatal dose of copper sulphate is:
A. 5-10 mgs B. 15-30 mgs
B. 5-10 gms D. 15-30 gms

223. Death in copper sulphate poisoning occurs mostly due to:
A. Cardiac arrest
B. Vascular collapse
C. Renal failure
D. Convulsions

224. Metal fume fever can be seen in poisoning by:
A. Arsenic B. Lead
C. Zinc D. Iron

225. Poison resembling viper snake bite is:
A. Ricin B. Crotin
C. Bhilawanol D. Abrin

217 C 218 D 219 B 220 A 221 A
222 D 223 C 224 C 225 D

226. Active principle used for the production of artificial bruise is:

A. Abrin
B. Bhilawanol
C. Crotin
D. Ricin

227. Pharoah's serpent is produced and burning a tablet of:

A. Mercuric cyanide
B. Mercuric chloride
C. Mercuric sulphide
D. Mercuric oxide

228. Most common type of poisonous snake in India is:

A. Cobra
B. Common krait
C. Russell's viper
D. Saw scaled viper

229. 3rd supraorbital shield touching eye and nasal shield is seen in:

A. Cobra
B. Krait
C. Viper
D. Sea snake

230. Vertically slit pupils are seen in:

A. Cobra
B. Krait
C. Viper
D. Sea snake

231. Cholinestrase is present in larger qualities in the venom of:

A. Cortalidae
B. Elapidae
C. Viperidae
D. Hydrophidae

232. Polyvalent anti-snake venom is prepared against the venom of:

A. Cobra, common krait and Russell's viper
B. Cobra, king cobra, common krait, saw scaled viper
C. Cobra, banded krait, Russell's viper and saw scaled viper
D. Cobra, common krait, Russell's viper and saw scaled viper

---

226 B 227 A 228 B 229 A 230 D
231 B 232 D

233. Bleeding from gums, rectum and site of bite is seen in bite by:

A. Cobra
B. Banded krait
C. Rusell's viper
D. Sea snake

234. Fatal dose of conc. sulphuric acid is about:

A. 5-10 ml
B. 15-20 ml
C. 25-30 ml
D. 35-40 ml

235. Antidote used in mineral acid poisoning is:

A. Sodium carbonate
B. Potassium hydroxide
C. Sodium bicarbonate
D. Magnesium oxide

236. Yellowish discoloration of stomach wall is seen in poisoning by:

A. Sulphuric acid
B. Nitric acid
C. Carbolic acid
D. Hydrochloric acid

237. Hypocalcemia is usually seen in poisoning by:

A. Carbolic acid
B. Salicylates
C. Oxalic acid
D. Ammonia

238. Leathery stomach is seen in poisoning by:

A. Sodium hydroxide
B. Cyanides
C. Copper sulphate
D. Phenol

239. Garlic-like smell can be detected in poisoning by:

A. Cyanide
B. Carbolic acid
C. Aluminium phosphide
D. Organophosphates

---

233 C 234 A 235 D 236 B 237 C
238 D 239 C

240. Greenish urine with albumin and traces of blood is seen on ingestion of:
A. Oxalic acid
B. Copper sulfate
C. Carbolic acid
D. Sheel's green

241. Antidote used in phosphorus poisoning is:
A. Copper sulphate
B. Dimercaprol
C. Pot. ferrocyanide
D. E.D.T.A.

242. Substance used for removing stains or used as bleach is:
A. Carbolic acid
B. Oxalic acid
C. Acetic acid
D. Acetyl salicylic acid

243. Substances used on the side of a safety match box include:
A. Pot. chlorate
B. Antimony sulphide
C. Red phosphorous
D. Yellow phosphorous

240 C 241 A 242 B 243 C

13

Medicolegal Procedures

FORENSIC OR LEGAL MEDICINE

It deals with application of medical knowledge for the solution of legal problems, e.g., in deciding cases of injuries, murder, sexual offences, poisoning, etc. The word Forensic is derived from Latin word, *forensis* which means *the forum* (belonging to the market place, a place of assembly).

TRIVIA
'The Father'
• Hippocrates: Medicine. • Paulo Zacchias: Legal Medicine. • Mathieu Orfila: Modern Toxicology. • **Prof. Jaising P Modi**: Forensic Medicine in India.
'The First'
• Medicolegal Expert: Imhotep. • Autopsy: Bologna, Italy by **Bartolomeo De Varignana**. • Book on Forensic Medicine: Italian, **Fortunato** Fedele.
In India
• First Medicolegal code: Manu Samriti. • The first medicolegal autopsy in India by Dr. Edward Bulkley. • The first Professor of Medical Jurisprudence Dr. CTO Woodford. • First Fingerprint Bureau: Kolkata, India by Sir William Herschel. • The Indian Medical Council was established in 1933. • The police system of crime investigation was introduced in India in 1861. • Coroners systems in 1871 in Bombay and Calcutta (no longer exist).

Inquest

- CrPC 174 deals with inquest.
- It is the investigation into the cause of death. Origin of Term – *Quaesitum: to seek.*
- It is conducted in cases of:
  - Murder.
  - Suicide.
  - Accidents; and
  - Suspicious deaths.

1. Police Inquest

- This is done by officer-in-charge of a police station.
- Medicolegal autopsy is ordinarily done on requisition of **sub-inspector of police** but not below the rank of **Head Constable.**
- The police officer visits scene of crime and prepares a report which includes description of wounds, the nature of weapon used and the apparent cause of death.
- The inquest report (**panchnama**) is then signed by the police officer and two witnesses. If foul play is suspected, body is sent for autopsy. **Sec. 179 IPC**–Refusal to Answer Police–Punishable.

2. Coroner's Inquest

No longer done in India.

3. Magistrate's Inquest

This is done by an Executive Magistrate (Collector, Deputy Collector, Tahsildar etc.) in cases of:

- Death in police custody.
- Death in mental asylum.
- Death due to police firing.
- Death in prison.

- Dowry death–Death of a woman within 7 years of marriage.
- Exhumation.

Magistrate's inquest is not conducted by, ***but can be ordered,*** judicial magistrate.

4. Medical Examiner's Inquest

- Medical examiner is a forensic pathologist, who conducts and supervise inquest.
- It is considered to be best form of inquest.
- It is prevalent in most of the states of USA.

Courts of Law

Types

1. Criminal.
2. Civil.

- **Criminal Courts:** These are of four types:
  1. **Supreme Court** is the highest court and has power of supervision over all courts in India.
  2. **High Court** is the highest court for the state. It may try any case and pass any sentence authorized by law.
  3. The **sessions court*** can pass any sentence authorized by law. It is **the lowest court which can pass death sentence**[NEET] but the death sentence passed by it must be ***confirmed by the High Court****.
     - An assistant sessions court can pass a sentence of imprisonment upto ten years.
     - Death sentence can be commuted by High Court, Supreme Court and President.
     - The sentence awarded by a court may be enhanced by the higher court.
     - Courts of trial–Magistrate and Sessions.
  4. **Magistrates are of three types: Sec. 29 CrPC 1973**
     a. **Chief Judicial Magistrate** can pass a sentence of imprisonment upto 7 years.

b. **First Class Judicial Magistrate** can imprison upto 3 years and fine upto 10 thousand rupees.
c. **Second Class Judicial Magistrate** can imprison up to 1 year and fine up to five thousand rupees.

- **Section 416 of CrPC**–A pregnant woman sentenced to death cannot be hanged till delivery and attainment of ***6 months of age*** by the child. **(Memorizer → 420 minus Four)**
- Types of **legal sentences** are–Death, imprisonment, fine.

Cognizable Offence (Grave Offence)

I. **Section 2 (c) CrPC:** Cognizable offenses or cognizable cases–Police officer can arrest without an arrest warrant, E.g., Murder, Rape, Dowry Death, Kidnapping, Theft, Criminal Breach of Trust, Unnatural Offences.
II. **Section 154** of CrPC provides, that under a cognizable offence, police officer has to receive the First Information Report (**FIR**) relating to the cognizable offence, which can be without the Magistrate's permission and enter it in the General Diary and immediately start the investigation.
III. If a cognizable offence has been committed, a police officer can investigate without the Magistrate's permission.

Subpoena or Summons [Sec. 61-70 CrPC] (Sub-Under, Poena-Penalty)

- It is **written legal document**NEET issued by the court and served on the witness under a penalty in all cases by the police officer to attend the court for giving evidence on a particular day and time.
  - Two types of subpoena:
    - **Subpoena *ad testificandum***→Attend and give evidence.
    - **Subpoena *duces tecum***→Attend, give evidence and bring documents specified along.

- If witness fails to attend the court, he may be fined or imprisoned in all types of summons, but he will be excused if he has a valid and urgent reason.
- Criminal courts have priority over Civil Courts.
- If witness is summoned by two criminal courts on the same day, he should give preference to higher court.
- If the summon is from 2 equal courts the preference is to be given to the summon received first.

Warrant (Sec. 70 CrPC)

A written order issued by a court after the filing of a complaint, but unlike summons, a warrant requires the police to arrest the person named in the warrant.

Conduct Money

- It is fee paid to a witness at the time of serving the summons to cover the expenses for attending the court.
- It is given only in **civil cases.**

Record of Evidence (Sec. 137 IEA)

The evidence of a witness is **recorded** as follows:

1. *Oath*

- Before giving evidence the witness has to swear by God or, solemnly affirm that he will tell the truth, whole truth and nothing but truth.
- It is compulsory and binds witness for evidence given.
- In oath-taking the witness has to keep his hand on a holy book. This does not apply to child below 12 years.*

Perjury– Sec 191 I.P.C.

It means **telling lies** by a witness under oath or failure to tell what he knows or believes to be true.

The witness can be prosecuted and punished for perjury **Sec 193 I.P.C.***

2. Examination-in-chief

- Questions are put to the witness by the lawyer who has summoned him.
- A **leading question** is one which includes the material facts and suggests to the witness, the answer desired and admits of a conclusive answer by YES or NO.
- Leading questions are **not** allowed.
  – ***Except when the witness is hostile.****

3. Cross-examination (139 IEA)

- The witness is questioned by the defence lawyer.
- **Leading questions are allowed.**
- The defence witness in a murder trial is cross examined by public prosecutor.

Questions to insult and annoy not allowed. *(Sec 152 IEA)*

4. Re-examination

- This is done by the lawyer, who has conducted examination-in-chief.
- Leading questions are **not** allowed.

5. Questions by Judge

Can be asked any time to clear his doubts.

Medical Evidence

Documentary Evidence

1. Medical Certificate

- They refer to disease, death, insanity, etc.
- Only a registered medical practitioner can give a valid certificate.
- If the patient dies, the doctor is legally bound to give death certificate without charging fees.
- If the doctor is not sure of the cause of death or, in cases of suspicion of foul play, the doctor should not give death certificate and the police should be informed.

2. Medicolegal Reports

- They are reports prepared by the doctor, usually in criminal cases, e.g., murder, assault, rape, poisoning, etc.
- They are admitted as evidence in court only when the doctor gives oral evidence on oath.

3. Dying Declaration (Sec 32 Indian Evidence Act)

- It is a written or oral statement of a person, who is dying due to some unlawful act, relating to the cause of his death.
- A magistrate should be called to record statement.
- If the condition of the patient is serious, the doctor or any other person can record the statement in the presence of two witnesses.
- The person need not take oath because it is believed that a dying person will not tell lies.
- Leading questions should not be asked.
- The signature of the declarant should be taken, and it should also be signed by the doctor and the witnesses.
- If the declarant survives, he is called to give oral evidence and the dying declaration becomes useless.

4. **Dying Deposition is Superior to Dying Declaration** because the accused has an opportunity of **cross-examination** the dying person, the person is under oath, the accused is present.

Dying Declaration	*Dying Deposition*
1. It can be recorded by Magistrate, Doctor, even a lay person.	1. It can be recorded only by the Magistrate.
2. The person is not put under oath.	2. The person is put under oath.
3. The person is not cross-examined.	3. The person is cross-examined.
4. Less superior to dying deposition.	4. Superior to dying declaration.
5. Accepted in India under Sec (**32 IEA**).	5. Not accepted in India.

5. Oral Evidence

- It is evidence which is given orally by a witness under oath in a court of law in connection with the case under inquiry.
- It is **more important than documentary evidence** because in this cross-examination can be done.
- **Documentary evidence** is accepted without oral evidence in the following conditions:
  – **Dying declaration.***
  – Expert opinion expressed in ***treatise***.
  – Evidence of a doctor recorded in ***a lower court***.*
  – Evidence given by a witness in a ***previous judicial proceeding***.
  – **Chemical examiner's report.***

Types of Witness

1. Common Witness

- He is a person who gives evidence about the facts observed by himself.
- Doctor is an ordinary as well as expert witness. He/She can volunteer the statement ***only if*** ordered to do so.

2. Expert Witness

- He is one who is qualified or experienced in a scientific or, technical subject and is capable of giving opinion from the facts observed by himself or others, e.g., doctor, fingerprint expert, handwriting expert, firearm expert, chemical examiner. **Oath is NOT necessary** in an expert opinion **expressed as a treatise**.

Doctrine of Res Gestae

- Res Gestae in Latin means "things done".
- This is the rule of law of evidence.

- It is admissible unlike Hearsay (non-admissible).
- Spontaneous declaration made by a person immediately after an event and before the mind has an opportunity to conjure a false story.

Vakalatnama: A document by which an advocate is empowered to appear before any court, on behalf of a party.

Writs: A writ is a formal written order issued by a court asking the addressee to refrain from or perform a specific act.

Five **Writs** as per Indian legal system:

I. ***Mandamus:*** Superior court asking a lower court to do or refrain from doing an action that is required by law.

II. ***Habeas Corpus:*** A court order that commands an **individual** or a government official who has restrained another to produce the prisoner at a designated time and place so that the court can determine **the legality of custody.**

III. ***Prohibition:*** **An extraordinary writ** issued by a higher court telling an inferior to keep within its jurisdiction.

IV. ***Quo Warranto:*** A writ restraining a person from holding a civil office to which he/she is **not entitled.**

V. ***Certiorari:*** A writ issued by the Supreme Court or High Court to **quash** the order already passed by an inferior court.

MCQs

1. Minimum age of a person, who can give consent for age determination is:

A. 12 **B.** 16
C. 18 **D.** 21

2. Conduct money is payable to:

A. A doctor for conducting autopsy
B. A witness for good conduct in the court
C. A witness in the civil court
D. A doctor for appearing in criminal court

3. Individual telling a lie under oath is:

A. Hostile witness
B. Professional liar
C. Charged with perjury
D. Professional misconduct

4. Open verdict in coroner's inquest means:

A. Verdict made known to the accused
B. Judgement made public
C. Case is kept pending
D. Case decided on previous judgement

5. Magistrate's inquest is held in following cases *except:*

A. Death in police custody
B. Dowry death
C. Death in jail
D. Death due to anaesthetic mishap

6. Punishment of imprisonment up to 3 years and fine up to Rs 5000.00 can be awarded by:

A. Chief Judicial Magistrate
B. Additional Sessions Judge
C. 1st Class Magistrate
D. 2nd Class Magistrate

1 A 2 C 3 C 4 C 5 D 6 C

7. Leading questions are permitted during:
A. Examination-in-chief
B. Cross-examination
C. Re-examination-in-chief
D. All of the above

8. Time limit for cross-examination is:
A. As long as examination-in-chief
B. Fixed by the presiding officer
C. Time available during that day
D. No time limit

9. Volunteering of statement is a privilege of:
A. Expert witness
B. Hostile witness
C. Common witness
D. None of the above

10. Who can record dying declaration?
A. Magistrate
B. Doctor
C. Police officer
D. All of the above

11. In case of death in lock up, the inquest is held by:
A. A Police Officer
B. A Magistrate
C. A Panchayat Officer
D. District Attorney

12. Which carries more weight in a court of law?
A. Dying declaration
B. Dying deposition
C. Both carry the same weight
D. Both are not significant

13. Dying declaration can be received by:
A. Medical Officer
B. Lawyer
C. Police Officer
D. All of the above

14. Dying deposition is recorded by:
A. Doctor
B. Magistrate
C. Police Officer
D. Lawyer

---

7 B 8 D 9 A 10 D 11 B 12 B 13 D 14 B

15. Who can be considered as an expert witness?

A. Medical men B. Firearm expert
C. Chemical examiner D. All of the above

16. Conduct money is paid to expert witness with summons from:

A. Civil Court B. Criminal Court
C. High Court D. Sub Magistrate

17. Perjury is:

A. Willful utterance of falsehood
B. An act committed within court premises
C. Failure to sign summons
D. Failure to appear as a witness

18. Death sentence can be awarded by:

A. First Class Magistrate
B. Second Class Magistrate
C. Sessions Court
D. Chief Judicial Magistrate

19. Which is a cognizable offence *except:*

A. Robbery
B. Murder
C. Rape
D. Attempted suicide

20. Medicolegal autopsy required the permission of:

A. Relatives
B. Medical Superintendent
C. Police
D. Magistrate

21. Which of the following is true about oath?

A. Not compulsory
B. Compulsory and binds witness for evidence given
C. Holds witness responsible for consequences of evidence
D. Witness is liable for prosecution if he does not take oath

15 D 16 A 17 A 18 C 19 D 20 C 21 B

22. A cognizable offence signifies:
A. Imprisonment upto 2 years
B. Imprisonment upto 3 years + Rs 1000 fine
C. Arrest without warrant
D. Only fine upto Rs 1000

23. An order for exhumation can be given by:
A. District Collector
B. Additional District Magistrate
C. Sub Collector
D. First Class Magistrate Only

24. Subpoena is a kind of:
A. Decomposed body tissue tribunal
B. Designation
C. Document
D. Court tribunal
E. Indelible ink

25. Medical certificate is:
A. Documentary evidence
B. Evidence
C. Hearsay evidence
D. Parole

26. The inquiry into the circumstances of death is called:
A. Homicide enquiry report
B. Inquest report
C. Open verdict
D. Adjourned verdict

27. An arrested person can request the magistrate for a medical examination of his body by a registered medical practitioner as per the following provision in the Code of Criminal Procedure:
A. Section 53
B. Section 54
C. Section 56
D. Section 57

22 C 23 D 24 C 25 A 26 B 27 B

28. In case of death in lock up, the inquest is held by:
- **A.** A Police Officer
- **B.** A Magistrate
- **C.** A Panchayat Officer
- **D.** District Attorney

29. Who can commute a death sentence?
- **A.** High Court
- **B.** Supreme Court
- **C.** President
- **D.** Any of the above

30. The sentence awarded by a court may be enhanced by the:
- **A.** Magistrate Court
- **B.** High Court
- **C.** Higher Court
- **D.** None of the above

31. Exhumation is usually done in the:
- **A.** Early morning
- **B.** Evening
- **C.** Night
- **D.** Any time

32. The time limit for ordering of exhumation in India is:
- **A.** 1 month
- **B.** 1 year
- **C.** 10 years
- **D.** No limit

33. A civil wrong is known as:
- **A.** Mutatis mutandis
- **B.** Pari passu
- **C.** Tort
- **D.** Ultra vires

34. The common type of inquest in India is:
- **A.** Coroner's inquest
- **B.** Police inquest
- **C.** Judicial magistrate's inquest
- **D.** Medical examiner's inquest

---

28 B 29 D 30 C 31 A 32 D 33 C 34 B

35. Perjury means giving willful false evidence by a witness while under oath, the witness is liable to be prosecuted for perjury and the imprisonment may extend to seven years. This falls under which section of IPC?

A. 190 of Penal Code
B. 191 of Penal Code
C. 192 of Penal Code
D. 193 of Penal Code

36. "Triage" is associated:

A. Warfare injuries
B. Road accidents
C. Gun shot injuries
D. Poisoning resuscitation

37. For exhumation the order should be passed by all *except:*

A. Chief Judicial Magistrate
B. Executive Magistrate
C. Police Officer
D. Sessions Judge

38. 20-year-old young female comes to a male gynaecologist for pelvic examination. The consent for examination is:

A. Implied consent
B. Written consent
C. Verbal consent
D. Informed consent

39. Dying deposition is more important than dying declaration because it is:

A. Made to a Magistrate
B. Oath is taken
C. Made in presence of accused
D. Cross-examination is permitted

35 D 36 B 37 C 38 A 39 D

40. After postmortem autopsy body is handed over to:

A. The authority who has conducted inquest in that particular case
B. Police station nearby
C. Coroner
D. Chief Magistrate

41. Perjury is:

A. Willful utterance of falsehood
B. Grievous injury
C. Contributory negligence
D. Criminal negligence

42. Exhumation can be done in India:

A. After 7 years
B. After 2 years
C. After 10 years
D. At any time

43. Which of the following statements about the award of capital punishment to a pregnant woman sentenced to death is correct? Death sentence cannot be carried out................. .

A. Until delivery
B. Until 6 months after the birth of the child
C. Until one year passes after the birth of the child
D. Until 2 years pass after the birth of the child
E. None of the above

44. Cross-examination of the prosecution witness is done by:

A. Public prosecutor
B. Defence counsel
C. None of the above
D. Judge

---

40 A 41 A 42 D 43 B 44 B

45. Perjury means:
A. Following the instructions of the jury
B. Violating the guidelines laid down by the jury
C. Giving false evidence after taking oath
D. Influencing the members of the jury

46. The power of Amnesty for capital punishment is vested with:
A. The President
B. Supreme Court
C. High Court
D. The Governor

47. After postmortem exam body has to be handed over to:
A. Investigating police officer
B. Relatives of victim
C. Magistrate
D. The civil authorities

45 C 46 A 47 A

14
Medical Jurisprudence

MEDICAL JURISPRUDENCE

It deals with legal responsibilities of the doctor concerned with the practice of medicine, e.g., medical negligence cases, consent, medical ethics, rights and duties of doctors etc.

MEDICAL ETHICS

- Deals with the moral principles, which should guide members of the medical profession in their dealings with each other, their patients and the state. Doctor ← → Patient.

  Medical Etiquette: Conventions governing Doctor ← → Doctor relationship.

Indian Medical Council Act, 1956

- The Indian Medical Council consists of medical practitioners elected from each state, each university and few nominated by Government of India.
- The **First Schedule*** of the Act contains the recognized medical qualification granted by universities in India.
  - The **Second Schedule*** those granted outside India.
  - **Third Schedule**

    Part I: Recognizes degrees by Indian Universities not included in 1st Schedule **(Memorizer: I→Indian)**.

For e.g.:
L.C.P.S.: Licentiate of the College of Physicians and Surgeons (CPS).

L.M.P.: Licensed Medical Practitioner.
(**Memorizer →** All Indian unusually sounding non-MBBS degrees come under Part I of Schedule Three).

Part II: Recognizes degrees by Foreign Universities not included in 2nd Schedule.

Indian Medical Council Functions

1. **Medical Register:** It maintains Indian Medical Register, in which names of all doctors who are enrolled on any State Medical Register are entered.
2. **Medical Education.**
3. **Recognition of Foreign Medical Qualifications.**
4. **Appeal Against Disciplinary Action:** If the name of any doctor is removed from the State Medical Register, he can appeal to the Central Government, which consults the IMC and gives decision, which is binding on the State Medical Council.
5. **Warning Notice** for serious professional misconduct.

Preservation of Medical Records of Patients

- **As per CoPRA:** Consumer (Patient) can file a complaint till 2 years after the service (Treatment) was provided.
- **Doctors** need to preserve records **for 3 years (Inpatients).**
- **Government Hospitals**
  - For Inpatient Case Sheets: 10 years.
  - For Medicolegal Registers: 10 years.
  - For outpatient records: 5 years.

State Medical Council

- They are autonomous bodies consisting of members elected by medical practitioners and those nominated by the state government.

- **Functions**
  1. *Medical Register:* The council appoints a Registrar who keeps a Register of medical practitioners, known as State Medical Register.
  2. *Disciplinary Control:* It has the power to remove the names of medical practitioner permanently or, for a specific period from the Register, if after an inquiry the doctor is responsible of serious professional misconduct. It can also re-enter the name so removed.
  3. They can issue warning notices.
- **Erasure of Name**
  1. The doctor's name is removed from the Medical Register.
     - If the entry is made wrongly or, as a result of fraud.
     - Penal erasure (Professional death sentence)*– If the doctor is guilty of severe professional misconduct. The doctor loses all the privileges of a registered practitioner.

Serious Professional Misconduct (Infamous Conduct in Professional Respect)

- It is any conduct of the doctor, which is considered as disgraceful or dishonorable. The conduct of the doctor is judged by medical practitioners of good repute and competence.

Warning Notice

- The following are some of the offences contained in the warning notice:
  1. Adultery (Voluntary sexual intercourse between a married person, and a person married or not, other than his or her spouse).
  2. Conviction by Court of Law.
  3. **Issuing false certificates (Sec. 197 IPC).**
  4. Performing criminal abortion or illegal operation.
  5. **Dichotomy or fee-splitting**, i.e., receiving or giving commission to professional colleague or

a manufacturer or trader in drugs or appliances, or a chemist, dentist etc.

6. **Covering**[NEET], i.e., assisting some person who has no medical qualification to attend, treat or perform an operation on some person.
7. **Advertisement:** Repeated advertisement in a newspaper by a medical practitioner is an example of **ethical negligence.**
8. '6' As for Warning Notice:
   - Association.
   - Addiction.
   - Alcohol.
   - Advertising.
   - Adultry.
   - Abortion (Unlawful).

Professional Secrecy

- The doctor obliged to keep secret all things about his patient, which he comes to know during his professional work.
- Professional secrecy may be divulged by demand of the court.
- The secrets regarding a patient can be revealed for:
  1. Protection of individual.
  2. Protection of the country.
  3. Interest of justice.

Privileged Communication

- It is a statement communicated by **a doctor to the concerned authority** to protect the interest of the community of state.
- Examples of privileged communication:
  1. A syphilitic bath in a public pool.
  2. Engine or bus driver found to be colour blind.
  3. A person with infectious disease working as a cook.
  4. A doctor's duty is to notify birth, death, and infectious disease to public health authority.

- Exceptions to the General Rule of Professional Secrecy is—**"CIVIC SIN"**:
  - **C** — **C**rime
  - **I** — **I**nfectious Disease
  - **V** — **V**enereal Disease
  - **I** — **I**nterest (Self)
  - **C** — **C**ourts of Law
  - **S** — **S**ervant and Employee
  - **I** — **I**nterest (Patients)
  - **N** — **N**egligence suits/Notifiable diseases.

Professional Negligence

- Medical negligence falls under following section – See 304A IPC, 312 IPC, 351 IPC.
- Professional negligence (malpractice) is the absence of reasonable care and skill, or willful negligence of a doctor in the treatment of a patient, which may result in injury or death.

1. *Civil Negligence:*

The following conditions should be satisfied to prove negligence **[4Ds]**.

- *Duty:* Existence of duty of care by the doctor.
- *Dereliction:* Failure of the doctor to maintain care and skill.
- *Direct causation:* Failure of the doctor to maintain care and skill.
- *Damage:* The damage which results must be reasonably anticipated.
  - Disclosure of professional secrets is a criminal offence in France, Germany.
  - Good plea for defence in a charge of malpractice.
    1. Absence of duty.
    2. Negligence of patient.
    3. The damage was unforeseen.
- **Res Ipsa Loquitor (R.I.L.)**

  i. It means the thing speaks for itself.

ii. This doctrine is applied both in civil and criminal negligence.

The rule is applied when following conditions are satisfied **"AXN"** is a memory aid for these conditions:

A — In **A**bsence of negligence injury would not have occurred.

X — Doctor had **X**clusive control.

N — Patient **N**ot guilty of Contributory **N**egligence.

The maxim of Res ipsa loquitor, is only a rule of evidence but that by itself cannot be used to determine the liability of negligence. Expert Medical Evidence is not required in R.I.L.

- **Novus Actus Interveniens (N.A.I.)**
  i. It means an unrelated action intervening and resulting in **Breaking the Chain**. Normally a person is responsible for his actions and also for its consequences. However, a new act intervenes (Act of God) which may result in diminishing the responsibility/liability of the original negligent individual.
  ii. This principle applies to cases of assault and accidental injury.

Medical Negligence vs. N.A.I.
Negligence by doctor —→Continuous Chain of causation leading—→ Injury to Patient (Doctor liable)
Negligence by doctor———X——**Novus Actus Interveniens—X—**breaks/severs the Chain of Causation → Injury to Patient (Doctor's liability diminishes. Defence against negligence)

2. Criminal Negligence

- It occurs when the doctor shows gross lack of competency, gross inattention, criminal indifference to the patient's safety, or gross negligence in the selection and application of remedies.

- **Gossypiboma** (also known as Textiloma or Cottonoid): A foreign object, such as cotton matrix or a sponge, left behind in a body cavity during an operation.
- It is practically limited to the cases in which patient has died.
- Sec 304 A IPC deals with criminal negligence.
- The doctor may be prosecuted by the police in a criminal court.
- The doctor can be punished with imprisonment up to two years.
- **Difference between Civil and Criminal Negligence.**

	Civil Negligence	*Criminal Negligence*
1. Offence	No clear and specific violation of the law need be proved	Must have specifically violated a criminal law in question
2. Negligence	Simple absence of care and skill	Willful, gross or culpable
3. Conduct of Physician	It is compared to a generally accepted simple standard of professional conduct	Not a single test
4. Trail by	Civil Court	Criminal Court
5. Consent for Act	Good defence	Not a defence
6. Punishment	Liable to pay damage	Imprisonment
7. Double jeopardy	Can be tried twice	Cannot be tried twice for same crime

Difference between Professional Negligence and Infamous Conduct:

	Professional Negligence	*Infamous Conduct*
1. Offence	Absence of care and skill or, willful negligence	Violation of code of medical ethics
2. Damage to person	Should be present	Need not be present
3. Duty of care	Should be present	Need not be present
4. Trail by	Courts–civil and criminal	State Medical Council

Contd.

Contd.

5. Punishment	Fine or imprisonment	Erasure of name or warning
6. Appeal	To higher court	To state or central government

Vicarious Liability (V.L.)

- An employer is responsible not only for his negligence but also for the negligence of his employees, if such negligence occurs in course of employment and within its scope, by the **principle of respondent superior*** (let the master answer). **Only Civil Responsibility**[NEET]. Surgeon and Anaesthetists are independent and do not come under the purview of V.L.

Contributory Negligence

- It is the negligence of the patient, combined with the doctor's negligence, which contributes to the injury as a direct cause and without which the injury would not have occurred. A defence for Civil Negligence; **not Criminal Negligence**.

Therapeutic Misadventure

- It is a case in which a patient is injured or dies due to some unintentional act done by a doctor or hospital.

DEFENCES available for a doctor against allegation of negligence.

Complete Defence

I. **Contributory Negligence (Only Civil Negligence**[NEET]**).**

II. **Volenti Non-Fit-Injuria**–To one who volunteers, no harm is done.

III. **Ex Turpi Causa:** If the patient who suffered damages while participating in a criminal activity, doctor is not responsible.

Other Defences

- Peer Acceptance Defence.
- Good Samaritans Defence: Rescue Cases or Emergency.
- Limitation → Statutory Limitation of 2 years.
- Therapeutic Misadventure.
- Res judicata which means – the **things** have been **decided**.
- Medical Mal-occurrence.
- Error in Judgment.
- Informed Consent.

Potential Q Zone

THE PEER ACCEPTANCE DEFENCE
Bolam vs. Bolitho Test (Medical Negligence) • **Bolam test:** This is based on the principle that a doctor does not breach the legal standard of care, and is therefore not negligent, if the practice is supported by a **responsible body of similar professionals.** • **Bolitho test:** A doctor cannot defend a case on the basis of a current practice by a responsible body of similar professionals that is **not reasonable or logical**. Bolitho legal test–modified, the 1957 Bolam test.

Some Other Legal Jargons

- ***Mutatis Mutandis:*** "With necessary changes being carried out, when comparing cases which are substantially same.
- ***Pari Passu:*** "With equal progress", i.e., Equitably without preference.
- ***Ultra Vires*:** Beyond the scope/power/authority.
- ***Tort:*** A civil wrong.

Euthanasia (Mercy Killing)

- It means causing painless death to a person suffering from hopelessly incurable and painful disease.

- Euthanasia advocates the administration of lethal doses of opium or other narcotic drugs. It has no legal sanction in India.
- First country to legalise euthanasia is **Netherlands.**

Consent Medical Practice

- Consent means voluntary agreement, compliance or permission.
  Section 13 of *The Indian Contract Act*: 'Two or more persons are said to consent when they agree upon the same thing in the same sense'.
- It may be:
  1. Express, i.e., specifically stated by the patient.
  2. Implied.
  3. Presumed consent is important in cases of emergency when consent cannot be taken.

Informed consent is an expressed consent which must contain four vital components **[C-I-A-S]. [Memorizer → C-I-A-S].**

1. Mental **Capacity** of the patient.
2. Complete **Information** to be provided by doctor.
3. Voluntary **Acceptance** of the procedure by the patient.
4. Should be person and the procedure **Specific.**

Reasons for Obtaining Consent

1. To examine, treat or operate upon a patient without consent is an assault in law.
2. If there is no informed consent the doctor may be sued for negligence.

Rules of Consent

- **Nuremberg Code of 1947:** The Nuremberg Code makes it mandatory to obtain voluntary and informed consent of human subjects. Consent is part of Medical Ethics.
- **Declaration of Helsinki** of World Medical Association 1964 emphasizes the importance of

obtaining freely given informed consent for **medical research.**

- **Doctrine of Paternalism:** It is a notion where the doctor takes up the role of a parent of the patient and starts deciding on behalf of the patient himself.
- **The principle of autonomy** is enshrined within **Art. 21** of the Indian Constitution, and is related with rules of consent.
  - **Doctrine of VOLENTI NON-FIT-INJURIA:** If an individual gives consent to suffer any harm or injury, he cannot claim damage for the same.
  - A woman should not be examined without her consent in medicolegal cases such as rape, pregnancy, abortion etc.
  - Doctor can examine a person, even by using reasonable force. If a person is arrested on a charge of committing an offence, and a sub-inspector of police gives requisition.
  - A prisoner should be treated without his consent.
  - Consent for an illegal act such as criminal abortion is not valid.
  - A person above **12 years** can give consent for **Non-Invasive Procedure,*** i.e., general physical examination.
  - A person above **18 years** can give consent for surgery **(Sec. 87 IPC).**
- Doctrine of Emergency and Consent: **Sec. 92 IPC.**
- A child below 12 years and an insane person cannot give valid consent.
- A consent given by a person under fear of injury or an intoxicated person is not valid **(Section 90 IPC).**
- Any harm caused to a person in good faith even without that person's consent is not an offence if the person cannot signify consent.
- An arrested person can be examined without consent if requested to do so by a police officer

not below the rank of a Sub-Inspector (**Section 53 IPC**).

- Consent of one spouse is **not necessary** for an operation (including MTP, where consent of husband not required) or treatment of another.
- For contraceptive sterilization consent of **both** husband and wife should be taken.

Exceptions to Consent

a. **Emergencies.**
b. **Knowledgeable waiver.**
c. **Therapeutic privilege:** Information can be withheld, when disclosure per se would be likely to cause harm to patients (e.g., when a patient with an unstable cardiac arrhythmia would have his or her situation exacerbated by the anxiety attendant on full disclosure of the risk of treatment). In emotionally disturbed patients the doctor should request a specialist consultation to establish that the patient is emotionally disturbed. The doctor should also note his decision in the patient's records explaining his intentions and the reasons for it.
d. **Incompetence:** Incompetent patients may not, as a matter of law, give an informed consent.
e. **Involuntary treatment:** This occurs most commonly when patients' refusals of treatment are specifically overridden following clinical, administrative, or judicial review.

Health Related Declarations of World Medical Association

1. Declaration of **Oslo**
   → Therapeutic Abortion
2. Declaration of **Sydney**
   → Definition of Death
3. Declaration of **Munich**
   → Discrimination in Medicine
4. Declaration of **Helsinki**
   → Human Experimentations and Clinical Trials

5. Declaration of **Lisbon**
   → Rights of Patients
6. Declaration of **Venice**
   → Terminal Illness
7. Declaration of **Tokyo**
   →Torture and Medicine
8. Declaration of **Geneva**
   → Modernized Version of Hippocratic Oath*
9. Declaration of **London**
   → International Code of Medical Ethics
10. Declaration of **Malta**
    → Role of Doctors in Hunger Strike
11. Protocol of **Istanbul**
    → Manual on Effective Investigation and Documentation of Torture

MCQs

1. **Professional death sentence is awarded by:**
   A. Medical Council of India
   B. Sessions Court
   C. State Medical Council
   D. Indian Medical Association
2. **Appeal against the punishment for professional misconduct is made to:**
   A. Medical Council of India
   B. High Court
   C. Health Ministry
   D. Indian Medical Association
3. **Moral principles, guiding dealing in the medical profession are known as:**
   A. Medical etiquette's
   B. Medical ethics
   C. Professional courtesy
   D. Medical norms
4. **Red Cross emblem can be used by:**
   A. Any person in medical services
   B. Any doctor
   C. Doctors in Government service
   D. Doctors in military service
5. **Professional negligence is failure on the part of a doctor for:**
   A. Wrong diagnosis
   B. Wrong treatment
   C. Absence of reasonable care
   D. Refusal to accept a patient

1 C   2 C   3 B   4 D   5 C

6. Doctrine of 'Res Ipsa Loquitur' can be applied in:
A. Prescription of overdose
B. Complications in an operation
C. Failure to achieve total cure
D. Contributory negligence

7. Contributory negligence is negligence by:
A. Doctor
B. Patient
C. Paramedical staff
D. Both by patient and doctor

8. Application of reasonable force to examine an individual without consent, is permissible in:
A. Accused of sexual assault
B. Victim of sexual assault
C. Pedestrian in road traffic accident
D. Psychiatric case

9. Usual punishment for criminal negligence by a doctor is:
A. Payment of damages
B. Imprisonment
C. Professional death sentence
D. Warning notice

10. Contributory negligence can be used as a defense in:
A. Civil negligence case
B. Criminal negligence case
C. Ethical negligence case
D. Departmental inquiry

11. At the time of registration the declaration made by a doctor is based on:
A. Declaration of Geneva (1948)
B. Declaration of Helsinki (1964)
C. Declaration of Tokyo (1975)
D. World Medical Associate Resolution (1981)

6 A 7 D 8 A 9 B 10 A 11 A

12. Functions of the State Medical Council include:

A. Maintenance of standard of medical education in the state
B. Disciplinary control of medical profession
C. Recognition of foreign medical qualification
D. Maintenance of health care system in the state

13. Standard of Medical Education in India is maintained by:

A. National Medical Board
B. Medical Council of India
C. Indian Medical Association
D. Directorate General of Health Service

14. Privileged communication can be made by a doctor in:

A. Notifiable diseases
B. HIV case
C. Malignant conditions
D. Divorce case

15. All the following are the conditions of defence available for a doctor against allegation of negligence *except:*

A. Medical maloccurrence
B. No fee for treatment charged
C. Therapeutic misadventure
D. Res Judicata
E. Error of judgement

16. Professional secrecy can be divulged:

A. If the doctor feels so
B. On demand by a court
C. Both of the above
D. None of the above

12 B 13 B 14 A 15 B 16 B

17. Law does not consider the following doctrine in a charge of criminal negligence:
A. Vicarious liability
B. Contributory negligence
C. Res ipsa loquitur
D. Novus actus interveniens

18. A quack gives a penicillin injection to a patient who dies due to it. Will the quack be relieved for his criminal responsibility by raising a plea of accident?
A. Definitely
B. Likely to
C. Never
D. Deserves to be acquitted on the strength of evidence

19. Disciplinary control over Registered Medical Practitioners is under:
A. State Medical Council
B. Indian Medical Council
C. Director of Medical and Health Services
D. Health Secretary of State Government

20. The following may be the examples of privileged communication *except:*
A. An impotent person marrying
B. A syphilitic taking bath in a public pool
C. Engine driver found to be colour blind
D. Pilot having hypermetropia

21. Criminal negligence is punishable under:
A. 306 IPC
B. 376 IPC
C. 304-A IPC
D. 304-B IPC

22. All of following can be used in criminal negligence *except:*
A. Res ipsa loquitur
B. Contributory negligence plea
C. Law of vicarious liability
D. Novus actus interveniens

17 A 18 C 19 A 20 A 21 C 22 C

23. Repeated advertisement in newspaper by a medical practitioner is an example of:
A. Infamous conduct
B. Ethical negligence
C. Criminal negligence
D. Privileged communication

24. Death of a patient due to an unintentional act by doctor, staff or hospital is:
A. Therapeutic misadventure
B. Vicarious liability
C. Therapeutic privilege
D. Diminished liability

25. Medical negligence falls under all *except:*
A. Sec. 304 A
B. Indian Contract Act
C. IPC 312
D. IPC 351

26. Normal courtesy of one doctor towards another is according to:
A. Medical etiquette
B. Medical ethics
C. Both of the above
D. None of the above

27. A doctor should not take fees for issuing certificate:
A. To a government employee
B. Death certificate
C. Poor patient
D. Psychiatric patient

28. In case of malpractice punishment is given by:
A. State Medical Council
B. MCI
C. IMA
D. High Court

29. Professional death sentence is:
A. Imprisonment for whole life
B. Rigorous imprisonment
C. Erasing the name from the panel of RMPs
D. None of the above

23 B 24 A 25 B 26 A 27 B 28 D 29 C

15

Medicolegally Important Sections/Acts

MEDICOLEGALLY IMPORTANT SECTIONS

Indian Penal Code

Section 44	Injury
Section 45	Life
Section 46	Death

Medicolegal Importance of Age

- Section 82. Act of a child under 7 years of age.
- Section 83. Act of a child above 7-12 years of immature understanding.
- Section 84. Act of a person of unsound mind/ **McNaughten's Rule.**
- Section 85. Act of a person incapable of judgment by reason of intoxication caused *against his will.*
- Section 86. Offence requiring a particular intent of knowledge committed by one who is intoxicated.

CONSENT

- Section 87. Act not intended and not known to be likely to cause death or grievous hurt, done by consent.
- Section 88. Act not intended to cause death, done by consent in good faith for person's benefit.

- Section 89. Act done in good faith for benefit of child or insane person, by or by consent of guardian.
- Section 90. Consent known to be given under **fear or misconception. FEAR**
- Section 92. Act done in good faith for benefit of a person without consent. **GOOD FAITH**
- Section 191. Definition and Section 193 Punishment of perjury (Punishment up to 7 years).
- Section 197. Issuing or signing false certificate.
- Section 201. **Causing disappearance of evidence of offence, or giving false information to screen offender**. (In a medicolegal case, **conducting embalming before autopsy** invites liability Section 201).
- Section 202. Intentional omission to give information of offence by person bound to inform.
- 269 IPC. Negligent act likely to spread infection or disease dangerous to life (**Nine→Negligence**).
- 270 IPC. Malignant act likely to spread infection or disease dangerous to life.

Offence Affecting Human Body

Section 299 to Section 377

299.	Culpable homicide
300.	Murder ←
301.	Culpable homicide by causing death of person other than person whose death was intended
302.	Punishment for murder
303.	Punishment for murder by life-convict
304.	Punishment for culpable homicide not amounting to murder
304A.	Causing death by negligence
304B.	Dowry death ←
305.	Abetment of suicide of child or insane person
306.	Abetment of suicide ←
307.	Attempt to murder ←
308.	Attempt to commit culpable homicide
309.	Attempt to commit suicide

AIIMS Nov. 11

Sections Related to Criminal Abortion

- Section 312 to Section 316

Section	Deals with
312 IPC With*	• Causing illegal miscarriage **with*** woman's consent
313 IPC	• Causing **illegal miscarriage without woman's consent**
314 IPC	• **Death of mother** caused **by act done with intent to cause miscarriage**
315 IPC	• Act done with **intent to prevent child being born alive** or to **cause it to die after birth**
316 IPC	• **Causing death of quick unborn child** by act amounting to culpable homicide

Abandonment of Child under 12 Years
- Section 317

Concealment of Birth
- Section 318

Hurt

Section 319

Grievous Hurt

- Section 320

319 IPC	• Definition of Hurt (whoever causes bodily pain, disease, or infirmity to any person is said to cause hurt)
320 IPC	• Grievous hurt definition
321 IPC	• Voluntarily causing hurt
322 IPC	• Voluntarily causing Grievous hurt
323 IPC	• Punishment for voluntarily causing hurt
324 IPC	• Voluntarily causing **hurt by dangerous weapons** or means
325 IPC	• Punishment for voluntarily causing grievous hurt
326 IPC	• Voluntarily causing **grievous hurt by dangerous weapons** or means
330 IPC	• Voluntarily causing hurt to extort confession or to compel restoration of property
331 IPC	• Voluntarily causing grievous hurt to extort confession or to compel restoration of property

Assault

- Section 351

Assault to Outrage the Modesty of Women

- Section 354

Rape

Definition Section 375
Punishment Section 376
[Section 228A. Disclosure of identity of the victim of certain offences etc like Section 376]

Unnatural Sexual Offence

Section 377

Death Sentence of a Pregnant Woman (Postponed or Commuted)

Section 416

Adultery

Section 497

Criminal Procedure Code (Cr.PC)

MEDICAL EXAMINATION

Cr.PC **53. Examination of accused** by medical practitioner at the request of police officer.

53a. Examination of person **accused of rape** by medical practitioner.

53. Accused of Rape.*

54. Examination of arrested person by medical practitioner **at the request of the arrested person**.

SUMMON (Section 61-70)

Cr.PC 61. Form of summons.
62. Summons how served.
64. Service when persons summoned cannot be found.
68. Proof of service in such cases and when serving officer not present.
69. Service of summons on witness by post.
70. Form of warrant of arrest and duration.

INQUEST

Cr.PC Section 174 Police Inquest.
Section 176 Magistrate's Inquest.
Section 293 Exception to Oral Evidence **(NOT Indian Evidence Act).**
Section 327
1. OPEN Trial.
2. **CLOSED Room, in camera trial in Rape cases.***

Indian Evidence Act

IEA Section 32 Dying Declaration.
Section 45 Expert Witness (Doctor is called in MLCs as expert witness).

Presumption

IEA Section 107 Presumption of Survivorship (SEVEN–Survive).
Section 108 Presumption of Death.

Related to Rape Law

IEA **Section 114 A:** Doctrine of Adverse Inference: When the victim states that she did not consent, the presumption is usually in her favour.

- **Chapter X of IEA – Of the examination of witnesses (135-166)**
  - **139. Cross-examination of person called to produce a document.**
  - **141. Leading questions.**
  - **152. Question intended to insult or annoy.**
  - **159. Refreshing memory.**
  - **162. Production of document.**

MEDICOLEGALLY IMPORTANT ACTS

1. **Drugs and Cosmetics Rules 1945**
   (Framed under: Drugs Act, 1940)
   - **Classification of drugs in schedules:**
     - C–Biological and special products.
     - E–Poisons.
     - F–Vaccines and Sera.
     - G–Hormonal preparations.
     - H–Drugs/poisons to be sold prescription of RMP.
     - J–Diseases for cure of which no drug should be advertised.
     - L–Antibodies, antihistaminic, chemotherapeutic agents.

2.	**Employees State Insurance Act**	**1948**
3.	**Indian Medical Council Act** **Schedule 1—India** **Schedule 2—Outside India**	**1956**
4.	**The Medical Termination of Pregnancy Act**	**1971 (Amend 1975)**
5.	**The Narcotic Drugs and Psychotropic Substance Act**	**1985**
6.	**Consumer Protection Act**	**1986**
7.	**Mental Health Act**	**1987**
8.	**Organs Transplantation of Human Act**	**1994**
9.	**Prenatal Diagnostic Technique Act**	**1994 (Amend in 2000)**
10.	**Delhi Anatomy Act**	**1953**

- The hospital authority can utilize **an unclaimed body** (a person who dies in hospital, prison or public places, which has not been claimed by any of his near relatives or personal friends within the prescribed timeline **of 48 hours**).
- Dead body is declared **unclaimed for the purposes of organ retrieval after 48 hours** as per the Transplantation of Human Organs Act 1994 (Act No. 42 of 1994).
- **As per the Police Manual** the dead body is declared unclaimed **only after 72 hours.**
- **In Road Traffic Accident,** body is declared **unclaimed only after 72 hours.**

11. **Clinical Establishments (Registration and Regulation) Act, 2010 –** To regulate all clinical establishments in India.
12. **Add more on our own !! (Potential Q Zone).**

16

Questions vs. Concepts

*"Examiners can fiddle with MCQs, choices, even Exam-pattern but they cannot fiddle with **the Concepts.**" – s.s*

- ***Latest Questions from: AIIMS; AIPG; Delhi PG, PGI; NEET.***
- ***Evergreen Concepts from Forensic Medicine.***

1. Autopsy was performed on a case of accidental death which shows two linear parietal fractures joining in midline. Which rule is used to determine that which fracture line has occurred before the second one?

A. Young's rule
B. Puppe's rule
C. Ashley's rule
D. McNaughten's rule

Concept:

Puppe's rule of Fracture Lines states that **an extending fracture line will cease** if it meets a preexisting fracture or suture line. In cases of Multiple Gun shot injuries **sequence of shots** may be deduced using Puppe's Rule.

But why other 3 choices cannot be the answer?

Ashley's rule of 149 is used for sexing sternum. Male > 149 mm, Female < 149 mm (outdated generalisation, cannot be relied on).

McNaughton's Rule also known as Legal Test and Right or Wrong Test : Daniel McNaughton's

1. B

trial for murder in 1843 led a jury to find him 'not guilty on the grounds of insanity'. McNaughton's Rule forms the basis of Sec. 84 of IPC, which deals with Criminal Responsibility of Insane. **Unsoundness*** of Mind – not criminally responsible.

Young's rule is a rule for evaluating the dosage of medicine for a child by adding 12 to the child's age, and dividing the sum by the age of the child, then dividing the adult dose by the result obtained. (Assignment–Google, **Clark's rule** !! it's potential Q).

Adult Dose × (Age ÷ (Age+12)) = Child's Dose

2. Which acid does not cause coagulative necrosis?

- **A.** HF (Hydro Fluoric* Acid)
- **B.** HCl
- **C.** HNO_3
- **D.** H_2SO_4

Concept:

- **HF is a weak! But Dangerous Atypical Acid.** (Weak Acid means ***Alkalish!*** And Alkalies are more dangerous).
- **Why HF is an exception?**
- HF's unique ability to penetrate tissue can cause **systemic toxicity** hence exposure to this acid should be treated with extreme care.
- **Unique Acid** to **penetrate tissue** because of high electronegativity of the fluoride anion.
- It is a weak acid (**Alkalish!**) which exists predominantly in the undissociated state compared to other acids. Once inside the

---

2. A

tissue the F anion is able to dissociate and **cause liquefactive necrosis** of soft tissue, bony erosion, as well as extensive electrolyte abnormalities by binding **the cations Ca^{2+} and Mg^{2+}.**

- **It causes hypocalcemia and hyperkalemia.**

(cf. → Typical acids **cause damage via the free H cations** resulting in **coagulative necrosis and poor tissue penetration).**

3. **Smell in shoe polish is because of:**
   A. Mercaptans
   B. Paraldehyde
   C. Nitrobenzene
   D. Aniline

Concept:

The Nose Knows! Box

• **Burnt Rope** Marijuana Opium • **Hospital Smell** Phenol Creosote • **Fruity** o Nitriles, Nitrites o Isopropyl alcohol o Ketoacidosis and Ketones o Ethanol, Isopropanol o Chloroform **ACRID** o Paraldehyde o Chloral hydrate • **Garlic** o Phosphorus o Arsine gas o Selenium o Thallium • **Musty–Fish or Raw Liver** • Zinc phosphide • Aluminum phosphide • Aniline	• **Hay** —Phosgene • **Mint** Methyl salicylate (Wintergreen) • **Mothballs** Naphthalene, Camphor, p-dichlorobenzene • **Pear** —chloral hydrate • **Pepper** — Tear Gas (o-chlorobenzylidene malonitrile) Pine oil • **Rotten eggs** — Hydrogen sulfide (can cause Olfactory fatigue, sparing the victim) — Carbon Disulfide — Mercaptans — Disulfiram — N-acetylcysteine • **Shoe polish** — Nitrobenzene • **Cigarette Packet Smell** —Nicotine • **Vinegar** — Acetic acid — Hydrofluoric acid

3. C

4. **Boiled lobster syndrome is seen in poisoning of:**
   - **A.** Hydrochloric acid
   - **B.** Chromic acid
   - **C.** Nitric acid
   - **D.** Boric acid

Concept:

Boric Acid Poisoning

- Boric acid is used as an Antiseptic, Cockroachicide!
- Severe poisoning can lead to **Beefy Red** skin rash, affecting palms, soles, buttocks and scrotum, characterized as a **Boiled Lobster Appearance.**
- The intense erythema is followed by desquamation and Extensive exfoliation. Looks like SSSS–**Staphylococcal Scalded Skin Syndrome.**
- **Red Velvet Mucosa is seen in Arsenic***

5. **Husband had some delusion of infidelity, because of which he throws Sulphuric Acid on wife. She was presented to emergency and died of burns. Which of the following is NOT SEEN in the chemical burn of the face of the wife?**
   - **A.** Absence of singing of hair
   - **B.** Presence of red line of demarcation
   - **C.** Burn at lower level to where acid falls
   - **D.** Presence of ulcerated patch

Concept:

Burns from corrosive substances show ulcerated patches and may be free from blisters, hairs are not singed in chemical burns and red line of

4. D 5. B

demarcation is absent. Strong acids produce dark leathery burns upon skin and leads to Coagulative Necrosis. Strong alkalis cause the skin to slough and leave moist, slimy and grayish area. Hydrofluoric acid causes Liquefactive Necrosis of skin and tissue.

6. **Ashley's rule is used to determine which of the following?**
   A. Sex
   B. Age
   C. Stature
   D. Race
7. **20 years old married woman took Aluminum Phosphide to commit suicide. The doctor who performed autopsy** concealed this **information willingly from investigating authority. This is punishable under which section?**
   A. IPC 198
   B. IPC 193
   C. IPC 202
   D. CrPC 84

Concept:

More IPCs to remember.

Section 201 IPC

Causing disappearance of evidence of offence, or giving false information to save offender.

Section 202

Intentional omission to give information of offence by **person bound to inform (doctor).**

6. A 7. C

Section 203

Giving false information respecting an offence committed.

Section 204

Destruction of document or electronic record to prevent its production as evidence.

8. In a bomb blast, all injuries can occur *except*:
   A. Bruise
   B. Fracture
   C. Abrasions
   D. Laceration

See: Marshal's Triad.

9. Most common method of suicide in India is:
   A. Hanging
   B. Fall from height
   C. Poisoning
   D. Drowning

Factual Concept:

As per national crime record bureau 2014, incidence of suicides is as follows:

Hanging	–	42%
Poisoning	–	26%
Fire/self immolation	–	7%
Drowning	–	6%

10. Peter fired gunshot on Jack. Jack escaped with thigh injury with no significant injury. Peter is punishable under which IPC?
   A. 302 **B.** 304
   C. 324 **D.** 326

8. B **9. A** **10. C**

Concept:

S. 324 IPC: Voluntarily causing Hurt (**def. 319 IPC**) by Dangerous weapon or means (No significant Injury).

S. 326 IPC: Voluntarily causing **GRIEVOUS HURT (def. 320 IPC)** by dangerous weapon or means.

11. The "knot" in judicial hanging is mostly placed at:

A. Below occiput
B. Angle of mandible
C. Below the chin
D. Choice of hangman

Concept:

Submental knot is thought to be **more effective** and ensures a quicker death, side of neck under the **angle of jaw (Subaural knot) on the left** is the commonly used position in India for judicial hanging. The length of rope from the point of suspension is equal to the height of individual. There is a sudden drop, resulting in fracture and dislocation of Upper Cervical Vertebrae (Fracture **of C2 from C3,** rarely C3 and C4).

12. Postponement of capital sentence in case of a pregnant woman comes under Cr.PC:

A. 416 B. 417
C. 418 D. 415

Concept:

Section 416 of Cr.PC provides that a woman sentenced to death IF found to be pregnant, the High Court shall order the execution of the sentence to be postponed and may, if it thinks fit, commute the sentence to imprisonment for life.

11. B **12. A**

13. Acrid odor is seen in the poisoning of:

A. Carbolic acid
B. Ether
C. Nitrobenzene
D. Paraldehyde

Concept:

Paraldehyde is clear, colorless liquid with an unpleasant ethereal odor and an acrid nauseous taste. Death from paraldehyde poisoning is rare.

Treatment of paraldehyde poisoning:

- Gastric lavage with **Sodium Bicarbonate.**
- Calcium gluconate and dextrose IV.

14. In a car accident, driver and front passenger both died. Which of the following in postmortem examination will help to identify driver *except*?

A. Seat belt over left shoulder
B. Sparrow footmark on the head
C. Whiplash injury to spinal cord
D. Steering wheel impact

Concept:

Driver will have Seat Belt over Right Shoulder and NOT Left (Indian system of driving).

Injuries seen in Road Traffic Accident:

- **Dicing Injuries:** These are short, linear, angulated, incised injuries caused by the characteristic cubed fragments of shattered tempered glass.
- **Stretch lacerations:** These are superficial, serpiginous to linear, parallel tears in the skin in areas of excess stretching.
- **Avulsion pockets:** When a bumper impacts the lower leg of a pedestrian, the force can shear the skin and subcutaneous

13. D **14.** A

fat away from the muscles, resulting in a hemorrhagic space.

- **Bumper fracture:** This is a fracture that occurs when the leg is struck by a bumper, and it is most often seen in the lower leg. At higher speeds, a characteristic fracture (originally called a **Messerer fracture. This fracture is wedge shaped,** with the apex of the wedge pointing in the direction of force, whereas the base represents the direction from which the force came.

15. According to the Amendment Act 2013, the age for sexual consent is:

A. 16 years **B.** 18 years
C. 20 years **D.** 15 years

Concept:

The Criminal Law (Amendment) Act, 2013: The age of consent in India has been increased to 18 years, which means any sexual activity irrespective of presence of consent with a woman below the age of 18 will constitute statutory rape.

Section 370 of Indian Penal Code (IPC) has been substituted with new sections, 370 and 370A which deal with trafficking of person for exploitation. A new section, **376A** has been added which states that if a person committing the offence of sexual assault.

16. Which is NOT true about BLAST injuries?

A. Injuries due to burns or air blast
B. Force of explosion decrease rapidly
C. Force of explosion is directional
D. Abrasion, bruise and fracture are triad of explosion

15. B **16. D**

Concept:

Marshal's Triad of bruises, abrasions and puncture lacerations with tattooing of part of the body indicate bomb explosion (Not Fracture).

17. Rat hole is associated with which injury?

A. Postmortem artifact

B. Firearm

C. Razor blade

D. Animal bit

Intermediate range wound from shotgun, may result in wound of entry which is irregular with ragged margin (Rat-hole injury) with satellite perforation at the margin of the main defect.

18. Segmented blood in retinal blood vessels. Sign is:

A. Rokitansky sign

B. Tache noir sign

C. Kevorkian sign

D. Carvallo's sign

19. Sweating is absent in:

A. Heat syncope

B. Miner's cramp

C. Heat stroke

D. Heat exhaustion

Concept:

Heatstroke is defined typically as **Hyperthermia and Anhidrosis** associated with an altered sensorium. This is attributed to an impaired functioning of the heat regulating mechanism caused by failure of cutaneous circulation and sweating due to prolonged exposure to heat.

17. B **18.** C **19.** C

20. A person was advised by his Orthopedic to get regular dressing of his wound done. But the patient did not give much care. The patient visited after some time at which time the Orthopedic again advised regular dressing but dint do the dressing himself as he said he was busy. Finally the wound enlarged and the underlying bone developed osteomyelitis. Which statement is true?

A. Doctor not guilty under "contributory negligence"

B. Doctor guilty under "Last clear chance" doctrine

C. Doctor not guilty under avoidable circumstance

D. None

Doctrine of last clear chance: A principle of tort law which requires an individual to take **every action at hand** to avoid an accident where peril to another human being is otherwise imminent, "but doctor dint do the dressing himself as he said he was busy".

21. A man fell from 35 feet height. Eye witnesses say that he landed directly on his feet. Which of the following injuries will confirm this fact?

A. Ring fracture of foramen magnum + lumbar spine injury

B. Pond fracture of skull + cervical spine injury

C. Gutter fracture of skull + cervical spine injury

D. Depressed fracture of skull + cervical spine injury

20. B **21.** A

22. Triple based smokeless gun powder consists of:

A. Nitrocellulose + Nitroglycerine + Nitro guanidine

B. Nitrocellulose + Sulphur + Nitro guanidine

C. Nitro guanidine + Potassium nitrate + Nitro-glycerine

D. Nitro guanidine + Potassium nitrate + Charcoal

Concept:

Black gun powder–It consists of potassium nitrate 75%, Sulphur 10% and Charcoal 15%.

Use of Constituent:

- Potassium nitrate–Oxidising agent. [*Dermal Nitrate Test/Paraffin Wax Test/ Diphenyl Amine Test* * is done to detect presence of gun powder on hands of the person who has fired the gun].
- Sulphur–Increase density by acting as binding agent.
- Charcoal–Fuel. [**N.B.:** FG "Fine Grain" denotes the fineness of gun powder particles, more Fs quicker it will burn].

Smokeless

* Nitrocellulose (single base).

** Nitroglycerine and nitrocellulose (double base).

*** With nitro guanidine* (triple base) powder.

Gun **P**owder on blood stained clothing thus can be visualized by Infra**R**ed **R**ays. (**Memorizer→GP-Rs**).

---

22. A

23. A person keeps a man under his power and threatens him to assault or cause harm without any intention to kill comes under:

A. Section 44
B. Section 351
C. Section 319
D. Section 320

Concept:

Chapter 15 is dedicated to IPC/CrPC/IEA and various Acts.

24. Choking is seen in:

A. Revolver
B. Sporting rifle
C. Shotgun
D. Pistol

Concept:

a. **Calibre**
Calibre is the distance between two diagonally opposite lands used for only rifled firearms*.

b. **Bore of gun/Gauge of gun**
- Used only in context of shot gun.
- Number of balls/pellets of equal size and weight as can be made from 454 gms (1 pound) of lead*.
- Bore determines the size of pellets*.

c. **Choking** is a constricting device at the muzzle end of the **shot gun**.* The purpose of choking is to lessen the rate of spread of shot after it leaves the muzzle (**c.f.** choking in mechanical asphyxia).

---

23. B **24. C**

Paradox Gun*–When the muzzlc end of the shot gun is rifled it is called Paradox gun.

d. **Revolver**

- It has a cylindrical magazine situated at the back of the barrel, which is capable of revolving motion. **The empty cartridge remains inside revolver** (Revolver never ejects cartridges automatically*).
- The range of revolver is 100 m.

e. **Air rifle and Air pistol**

- In these, compressed air is used to fire lead sluds.
- Empty cartridges an ejected out from automatic pistol.

25. A police officer brings the aborted product of conception of size 2 cm and weight 10 gm. For all forensic purposes what will be the age of the fetus?

A. 2 weeks
B. 4 weeks
C. 6 weeks
D. 8 weeks

Concept:

Rule of Haase

A rough! method of calculating the age of the foetus.

1. **Upto 5 months**, age of foetus = √Length (in cm) [Under root of length].
2. **> 5 months** = (length (in cm)/5) = months (**Morrison's* modification of Hasse's Rule**).

High School Maths: Age in months = Under root of 2 = 1.44 Months = 4 × 1.44 weeks = 5.76 months ~ **6 weeks.** 1 Month = 4 weeks.

25. C

26. A woman assaulted by neighbor was brought to you in the emergency department with fracture of middle tooth. Injury was extended medially to the mouth and there was also contusion to bilateral leg. What is the nature of thc injury?

A. Grievous injury
B. Simple injury
C. Dangerous injury
D. Assault

Concept:

According to **S 320 I.P.C. (Only Defines*)** any of the following injury is grievous: The eight clauses of grievous injury can be remembered with the help of sentence:

"**E**very **S**tudent **H**as re**MEMBER**ed Injury's **D**efinition and **F**orgot it within **20 days** of **P**assing Exams" (To decipher please read Chapter 3).

Seventhly: Fracture or dislocation **of a bone or tooth. (Discontinuity till medullary cavity is considered grievous)**.

27. A young man with known history of heroine addiction is brought in the emergency in unconscious state by his friends. On examination his *pupil are pin point*. What will be the treatment of choice?

A. Oral naltrexone **B.** IV naloxone
C. Oral diazepam

Concept:

A. The preferred, more definitive treatment for the typical overdose is the narcotic **antagonist naloxone I.V.**

B. Chemical test to detect the presence of opium.

26. A **27. B**

- **MARQUIS TEST***
- **DENIGES' TEST**
- **HUSEMANN'S TEST**

C. **HEROIN** (Diacetyl Morphine):

- Also known as: Smack, Brown sugar, Junk, Dope.
- It is white in color.
- **"Cutting In":** Term used for adulteration of heroin.
- Substances used for adulterations:
  - Quinidine
  - Mannitol
  - Fructose
  - Talc
  - Chalk powder.
- Heroin + cocaine is called **"Speed Balls"**.

D. **Postmortem hypostasis:** Black colored (Heroin is illegal, available in **black** market leads to **Black** PMS).

E. **Constricted pupil–Miosis (to avoid confusion only remember one list either constriction or dilation).**

BCMOP

- Barbiturates
- Carbolic acid
- Chloral hydrate
- Morphine (opium)
- Organophosphorus poisoning
- Pontine hemorrhage

Add more yourself!

F. **What is Coma Cocktail?**

Combination of 3 medicines can be given in unknown poisoning with coma [remember **DNB**]

Dextrose (50%) 100 ml

Nalaxone 2 mg

$\mathbf{B_1}$(Thiamine) 100 mg.

28. In the forensic laboratory some samples are being examined under ultraviolet ray, the doctor notices blue white colour of the sample.

Which is the most probable content of the sample?

A. Semen **B.** Urine
C. Pus **D.** Leucorrhoea discharge

Concept:

Dried semen can be visualized using blue light, **ultraviolet light** (also known as Wood's Lamp), Semen will fluorescence due to the presence of molecules such as Flavin and Choline-conjugated proteins.

The color of this fluorescence will vary from **blue white to yellow**, depending on the light equipment used.

Confirmatory Tests for Semen

A. ***The Christmas Tree Stain.***

B. ***RSID–Semen Strip Test*** identifies the presence of the **seminal vesicle-specific antigen or semenogelin.**

C. ***Prostate Specific Antigen:*** Forensic labs utilize a **Glycoprotein** P30 test to screen for PSA. This test has replaced the quantitative analysis for acid phosphatase.

D. **MHS-S1** is also positive and a highly reliable test for semen.

E. **Lactate dehydrogenase (LDH) Isoenzyme** using Electrophoresis Method (**Absolute proof** of semen).

(Absolute proof of **sexual intercourse** is finding at least 1 unbroken sperm or LHD isoenzyme detection of sperm).

Presumptive Tests for Semen

A. **Visual Detection: Dried semen** can be visualized using blue light, **ultraviolet light** (also known as Wood's Lamp). Semen will

28. A

fluorescence due to the presence of molecules such as Flavin and Choline-conjugated proteins. The color of this fluorescence will vary from blue to yellow, depending on the light equipment used.

B. The Acid Phosphatase Test:

- The prostatic secretion element of seminal fluid contains a very much **higher** percentage of Acid Phosphatase (AP).
- **Brentamine spot test:** In the presence of **Alpha-Naphthyl acid phosphate and Brentamine Fast Blue,** AP will produce a dark purple color in less than a minute.
- Analyses of post-coital vaginal swabs show that AP activity will markedly decrease after 24 hours and diminish after 48 hours.

Classical Tests

a. **Florence test (Choline Per. Iodide Crystals): A negative test means the fluid is not semen.**

b. **Barberio's test:**
- In **Barberio's test**, presence of **spermine in semen** is detected.
- Spermine picrate crystals are seen.

c. **Creatine phosphokinase:** Level of CPK is high in seminal fluids, can be detected in old stains of 6 months.

d. **Ammonium molybdate test:** For semen stains, detect presence of phosphorous.

e. Serological typing of the semen is possible by **precipitin method**.

29. All of the following are true about methanol poisoning *except:*
- **A.** Fomepizole is a competitive inhibitor of aldehyde dehydrogenase
- **B.** Minimum lethal dose of methanol is 1.25 gm/kg body weight
- **C.** Formic acid is mainly responsible for toxicity
- **D.** Methanol causes snow field vision

30. Lateral traction test is done in unnatural sexual offences in:
- **A.** Habitual active agent
- **B.** Pedophilia active agent
- **C.** Bestiality active agent
- **D.** Habitual passive agent

Concept:

Characteristics of Habitual Passive Agent

- **Shaving of anal hair**, no bloodstains, **loose foreign hair** and **smears of lubricants.**
- **Perianal skin thickened** and **keratinized.**
- No **pain** or **tenderness during digital examination**.
- **Anal sphincter** is **lax, opening is patulous, canal is dilated**
- Loss of fine symmetric rugal pattern along with congested or dilated veins.
- **Lateral Traction Test: External anal sphincter relaxes as a reflex** when **bimanual traction is applied to the buttocks**.
- **Anal opening** is **more deeply situated** than usual due to absorption of subcutaneous fat giving a **funnel shaped depression of buttocks.**
- **Rectum: Thickened, congested** and **prolapse of mucosa with disappearance of radial fold.**

---

29. A **30. D**

31. According to "DELHI ANATOMY ACT 1957", a person died in road traffic accident, the dead body is said to be unclaimed after:

A. 24 hours **B.** 48 hours
C. 72 hours **D.** 96 hours

Concept:

- In a Road Traffic Accident, Delhi Anatomy Act 1957, will be read with Section 174 CrPC, as per police manual autopsy would be conducted after **72 hours** (unclaimed body).
- Dead body is declared unclaimed for the purposes of organ retrieval **after 48 hours** as per the Transplantation of Human Organs Act 1994 (Act No. 42 of 1994).
- As per the Police Manual the dead body is declared unclaimed only after **72 hours.**

32. Embalming without issuing death certificate is punishable under section:

A. IPC 201 **B.** IPC 297
C. IPC 299 **D.** IPC 498

33. Stack Formula is used to estimate age through dentition is for:

A. Infants
B. Adults 25-50 years
C. Adult >50 years
D. Elderly

34. DNA is best obtained from autopsy from which organ?

A. Liver
B. Kidney
C. Brain
D. Spleen

---

31. C **32. A** **33. A** **34. D**

Concept:

After discussion with some of the senior professors of Forensic Medicine, who confirmed that the answer key likely considered **Spleen** as the answer and cited the following reference from **Postmortem Technique Handbook By Michael T. Sheaff, Deborah J. Hopster.**

35. Palate print commonly taken from:

A. Anterior part of palate
B. Lateral wall of palate
C. Medial wall of palate
D. Posterior palate

Study of this method is advantageous because:

1. Prints (ridge pattern) do not change during growth.
2. It is protected from trauma due to its situation.
3. It is protected from heat by buccal pad of fat and tongue.
4. Even in twins, the pattern of rugosities may be similar but not identical.

36. Flaying seen in what type of lacerated wound?

A. Tear **B.** Shearing force
C. Avulsion **D.** Pressure

37. Which of the following is wrong?

A. 300–Murder
B. 304–Culpable homicide not amounting to murder
C. 306–Attempted suicide
D. 307–Attempt to murder

38. What is the Section under which punishment is given for issuing a false medical certificate?

---

35. A 36. C 37. C 38. D

A. IPC137 B. IPC147
C. IPC157 D. IPC197

39. Giving false evidence under Oath is defined under section:

A. 151 IPC B. 161 IPC
C. 181 IPC D. 191 IPC

40. 1st ossification centre appears at:

A. Beginning 2nd I/U month
B. Beginning of 3rd I/U month
C. End of 3rd I/U month
D. 4th month of gestation

41. According to organ transplantation Act 1994 what punishment for doctor if found guilty?

A. 2 years B. More than 5 years
C. 4 years D. 2-5 years

Concept:

There has been an amendment in Organ Transplantation Act in August 2011, where the punishment has been made more severe between 5 and 10 years

42. A chronic alcoholic - assaults neighbor - had quit drinking 4 days back - now has delirium tremens. He is:

A. Responsible for committing the crime
B. Not responsible under Sec 84 IPC
C. Partially responsible
D. Responsibility can't be fixed from the given history

Concept:

Drunkenness is never an excuse, but when drunkenness becomes a disease then it does become a defence. Delirium Temens is a disease so person is not responsible, under Sec. 84 (unsoundness of mind).

---

39. D 40. A 41. B 42. B

43. Condition promoting adipocere formation:
- **A.** Dry and hot
- **B.** Hot and humid
- **C.** Dry and optimum
- **D.** Humid and optimum (temperature)

44. What does the word "cardiac polyp" mean?
- **A.** Acute infarct
- **B.** Cardiac aneurysm
- **C.** Benign tumour
- **D.** Fibrinous clot

Cardiac Polyp: Mural thrombus in the right/left atrium at the time of postmortem examination appears as pedunculated mass with a stalk attached to wall of the heart and main mass in the lumen in cavity of the heart.

45. In civil negligence, onus of proof is with:
- **A.** Judicial first degree magistrate
- **B.** Police not below the level of sub inspector
- **C.** Doctor
- **D.** Patient

Doctrine of Burden of Proof

In criminal litigation, the **burden of proof is *always* on the state**. The state must prove that the defendant is guilty. The defendant is *assumed* to be innocent; the defendant needs to prove nothing. (There are exceptions. If the defendant wishes to claim that he/she is insane, and therefore not guilty, the defendant bears the burden of proving his/her insanity. Other exceptions include defendants who claim self-defense or duress.)

In civil litigation, the burden of proof is initially on the plaintiff (patient in case of Medical Negligence suit). However, there are a number of technical situations in which the burden shifts to the defendant. For example, when the plaintiff has made a prima facie case, the

43. D 44. D 45. D

burden shifts to the defendant to refute or rebut the plaintiff's evidence.

46. A man working as a pest killer comes to OPD with pain abdomen, garlic odour in breath and transverse Meis lines on nails. What is diagnosis?

A. Arsenic poisoning **B.** Lead poisoning
C. Mercury poisoning **D.** Cadmium poisoning

47. Formication and delusion of persecution occurs together in: (Repeat from AIIMS May 2009)

A. LSD (Purple Gaze)
B. Cocaine psychosis (White Lady)
C. Canabis
D. Amphetamine

Magnan's symptoms or cocaine bug is characteristic, in which there is feeling as if grains of sand are lying under the skin or some small insects are creeping on the skin (**tactile hallucinations**).

This phenomenon is also known as formication. Some subjects report hallucinations of weak flashes of light, termed **"snowlights"**.

Hunan's Hand – Severe Contact Dermatitis due to Capsicum.

Gunchi – Abrus Precatorius – Suis – Cattle Poison.

48. During autopsy, if spinal cord is to be examined what is the most commonly used approach?

A. Anterior` **B.** Posterior
C. Lateral **D.** Anterolateral

49. Degrees awarded by Indian universities are mentioned in:

A. Schedule I of MCI Act
B. Schedule II of MCI Act
C. Part 1 of schedule III
D. Part 2 of schedule III

46. A **47. B** **48. A** **49. A**

Recognition of Medical Qualification Granted by Universities or Medical Institutions in India

- The medical qualifications granted by any university or medical institution in India which are included in the **First Schedule** shall be recognised medical qualifications for the purposes of this Act.
- The medical qualifications granted by medical institutions **outside India** which are included in the **Second Schedule** shall be recognised. medical qualifications for the purposes of this Act.
- The medical qualifications granted by medical institutions in India which are not included in the **First Schedule** and which are included in **Part I of the Third Schedule** shall also be recognised medical qualifications for the purposes of this Act.
- The medical qualifications granted by medical institutions outside India, before such date as the Central Government may, by notification in the Official Gazette, specify which are included in **Part II of the Third Schedule** shall also be recognised medical qualifications for the purposes of this Act.

50. Sparrow marks are seen in:

A. Gunshot injuries
B. Stab injury of face
C. Vitriolage
D. Windshield glass injury

SparroW*–Foot Mark is bizarre laceration seen on face due contact with shattered W*ind-screen.

51. Which organ obtained from a cadaver is not used for transplantation?

A. Blood vessel **B.** Lung
C. Liver **D.** Bladder

50. D **51. D**

52. A patient presented to the casualty with bluish grey pigmentation of conjunctiva, mucous membranes, nails and tachycardia after ingestion of a poison. What is the poison?

A. Mercury **B.** Arsenic
C. Lead **D.** Copper

Answer should be Silver (Ag), if there was no silver in choice, then could be copper.

53. A poison which is illuminous, translucent, cylindrical and waxy?

A. Iodine
B. Ammonium bromide
C. Cobra venom
D. Yellow phosphorous

54. Autorickshaw ran over a child's thigh, there is a mark of the tyre tracks, it is an:

A. Contact bruise
B. Patterned bruise
C. Imprint abrasion
D. Ectopic bruise

55. Rave drug is:

A. Cannabis **B.** Cocaine
C. Heroin **D.** Ecstasy

Ecstasy (MDMA)

Street names: XTC, X, E, Adam, The hug drug, The love drug.
Method of ingestion: Orally.
Appearance: Various colors and shapes usually in tablet or capsule form.
Effects: Pupil dilation, inattention, increased vitals, hyperactivity, increased body temperature, sweating profusely or not, bruxism, muscle cramping, trisma, teeth grinding, nausea, hallucinations, blurred vision, paranoia, depression.

52. D 53. D 54. C 55. D

Negatives: Hyperthermia (water toxicity) can be fatal and is the leading cause of death. Can kill with first use, rapid tolerance, extreme depression.

56. All are true about world health report 2008 *except*:

A. Social reforms
B. Leadership
C. Polices
D. Economic reforms

57. Signature fracture refers to:

A. Depressed skull fracture
B. Suture displacement fracture
C. Contrecoup injury
D. Fracture at foramen magnum

58. Child brought to casualty with reports of violent shaking by parents. Most likely injury is:

A. Long bone fracture
B. Ruptured spleen
C. Subdural hematoma
D. Skull bone fracture

Concept:

The term "whiplash shaken-baby syndrome" was coined by Caffey to explain this constellation of infantile subdural and subarachnoid haemorrhages, traction-type metaphyseal fractures, and retinal haemorrhages and was based on evidence that angular (rotational) deceleration is associated with cerebral concussion and subdural haematoma (being the MOST CHARACTERISTIC FEATURE of violent shaking of an infant by the parent).

59. Gun powder on clothing can be visualized by:

A. Magnifying lens
B. UV rays
C. Infrared rays
D. Liquid spray/solution spray

---

56. D **57. A** **58. C** **59. C**

60. Which of the following is used in rape victims to determine of rupture of hymen and whether rupture is recent or old?
A. Gaba rod
B. Gram rod
C. Cylinder rod
D. Glaister Keen rod

61. Autorickshaw ran over a child's thigh, there is a mark of the tyre tracks, it is an:
A. Contact bruise
B. Patterned bruise
C. Imprint abrasion
D. Ectopic bruise

Concept:

Imprint or patterned abrasions may result from forceful impact, as in a pedestrian struck by a vehicle. The importance of patterned abrasions lies in the fact that their shape can be matched to the causative object, and for this reason they should be documented by photography with a scale, or by an accurate tracing. Common examples of imprint abrasions are the sole patterns of footwear in kicking assaults, and motor vehicle tyre tread marks in run-over pedestrian deaths. **Patterned bruise takes place rarely in exceptional cases, when there is death after the injury.**

62. Aluminum phosphide poisoning—all true *except*:
A. Sub-endocardial infarcts
B. Produces phosphine gas
C. Oesophageal stricture
D. Cyt. A oxidase inhibitor

60. D **61.** C **62.** D

Concept:

Aluminum phosphide (Celphos) toxicity appears to be due to release of **PHOSPHINE** on contact with moisture. This phosphine gas due to non-competitive inhibition of **cytochrome C oxidase system** of mitochondria or damage by free radicals causes global hypoxia. Organs with the greatest oxygen requirements appear to be especially sensitive to phosphine, including the brain, kidneys, heart and liver. Phosphine has a characteristic odor described as "decaying fish". Cardiac Dysrhythmias probably secondary to electrolyte imbalances have been described in sub-lethal acute exposures. Transient atrial fibrillation and **subendocardial infarction, adrenocortical injury** with elevated serum cortisol levels have been reported.

63. True about subendocardial hemorrhage are all *except:*

A. May be seen after head injury
B. Involves RV wall
C. Continuous pattern
D. Flame shaped hemorrhages

Concept:

Subendocardial hemorrhage are found after intracranial hemorrhage following injury due to trauma, suddenly hypotension following any bleeding problems, obstetric complication, toxic poisoning particularly with **iron, arsenic, cocaine and cerebral hemorrhage strokes**. SEH involves **left** ventricular walls, flame shaped confluent, non-petechial and continuous. SEH are signs of agonal vital events. **(Page 295, Forensic Pathology Reviews: Michael Tsokos)**

64. Spanish WINDLASS technique is a form of which type of execution?

A. Garroting **B.** Mugging
C. Bansdola **D.** Hanging

63. B 64. A

65. Pale infarct not seen in:

A. Kidney **B.** Spleen
C. Heart **D.** Lung

Concept:

Anemic infarcts (also called **white infarcts**) are white or pale infarcts caused by arterial occlusions, and are usually seen in the heart, kidney and spleen. These are referred to as "white" because of the lack of hemorrhaging and limited red blood cells accumulation (compare to hemorrhagic infarct). The tissues most likely to be affected are solid organs which limit the amount of hemorrhage that can seep into the area of ischemic necrosis from adjoining capillary beds. The organs typically include single blood supply (no dual arterial blood supply or anastomoses).

66. Wid marks formula:

A. Alcohol
B. Time since death
C. Time since injury
D. Identification

Concept:

In order to calculate the **Blood Alcohol Concentration**, we must divide the weight of the alcohol by **the weight of only the portion of the body that holds the alcohol,** rather than the weight of the whole body. Widmark's original research, still valid today, found that the average man's body can hold alcohol in even distribution in **68% of its weight**. Widmark called this "0.68" factor his Widmark 'r' factor. The lower case "r" stands for "reduced body mass", or "reduzierte körpermasse".

65. D **66. A**

67. **A 20-year-old boy is having diarrhea, rhinorrhea, sweating, what is the most probable diagnosis?**
A. Cocaine withdrawal
B. Heroin withdrawal
C. Marijuana withdrawal
D. LSD withdrawal

Concept:

Heroin withdrawal symptoms: Restlessness, insomnia, diarrhea, vomiting, cold flashes with goose bumps, kicking movements, muscle and bone pain.
Cocaine withdrawal symptoms (cocaine crash): Fatigue, depression, restless behavior and a feeling of anxiety or paranoia.
Marijuana withdrawal: Irritability, anxiety, physical tension, increased aggression/anger, strange dreams.
LSD withdrawal: For LSD, the term **withdrawal** does not have the same meaning as for drugs that are habit-forming or addictive. While LSD use can rapidly lead to tolerance, it is not addictive.

68. **About cranial trauma false is:**
A. Racoon eyes seen in subgaleal hemorrhage
B. Depressed skull fracture is always over the immediate area of impact of brain
C. Corticocavernous fistula occur in base skull fracture
D. Post traumatic epilepsy seen in 15%

Concept:

Rule of Thumb*: "Always" and **"Never"** in choices, most of the time correct answer.
*Apply at your own risk.

- **BATTLE SIGN**–Bruising behind ear at mastoid region, due to petrous temporal bone fracture (middle fossa fracture).

67. B **68. B**

- **LIGHT HOUSE SIGN**–Seeping out of secretions in acute OTITIS media.
- **RACOON SIGN**–Indicate subgaleal hemorrhage, and not necessarily base of skull fracture.
- **STANKIEWICK'S SIGN**–Indicate orbital injury during FESS. Fat protrude into nasal cavity on compression of eyeball from outside.
- **TEA POT SIGN** is seen in CSF rhinorrhoea.

69. The age of a 15-year-old female is best determined by the radiograph of:

A. Lower end of radius and ulna
B. Upper end of humerus
C. Upper end of radius and ulna
D. Xiphisternum

Concept:

Joints	*Approximate age of fusion*
Shoulder joint	18 years
Elbow joint	16 years
Wrist joint	18 years
Hip joint	17-18 years
Knee joint	18 years
Ankle joint	16-17 years

70. Sodium fluoride is used for preservation:

A. Urine **B.** Blood
C. Alcohol **D.** Carbonic acid

Concept:

- NaF should be added to urine, blood, vitreous humor for alcohol estimation and to samples of:

- Cocaine (C).
- Carbon monooxide (C).
- Cyanide (C).

71. Maximum congestion is seen in:

A. Choking
B. Hanging
C. Strangulation
D. Drowning

72. In fresh water drowning the death occurs within 4-5 minutes of submersion due to ventricular fibrillation. Which of the following reasons is responsible for this?

A. Total asphyxia produced due to fresh water
B. Laryngospasm causing vagal inhibition
C. Haemoconcentration of blood caused by the osmotic pressure effect
D. Haemodilution, overloading of heart and haemolysis resulting in release of potassium

Concept:

Drowning in Fresh Water

- Death in fresh water drowning in comparison to salt water is earlier.
- Drowning in fresh water leads to haemolysis and haemodilution, hyperkalemia and the cause of death is ventricular fibrillation.
- In fresh water drowning, chloride content of the left side of the heart is 50% lower.

73. Bevelling of the skull is seen in the:

A. Broad end of the entry point in bullet injury
B. Narrow end of the entry point in bullet injury
C. Exit point of bullet
D. Depressed fracture of the skull

Concept:

Bevelling of the skull in bullet injury: The principle which guides the occurrence of

71. C 72. D 73. C

bevelling is that the bullet produces bevelling in the second layer (or exit point).

- In entry wound the bevelling is present in inner table of skull.
- In exit wound the bevelling is present in the outer table of skull.

74. All are components of black gun powder *except*:

A. Sulphur **B.** Charcoal
C. Potassium nitrate **D.** Lead peroxide

Concept:

- **Black gun powder**–It consists of potassium nitrate 75%, sulphur 10% and charcoal 15%.

75. When a group of muscles of a dead body were in state of strong contraction, immediately prior to death and remain so even after death, the condition is termed as:

A. Gas stiffening **B.** Rigor mortis
C. Cadaveric spasm **D.** Cold stiffening

Concept:

Cadaveric Spasm or Instantaneous Rigor or Cataleptic Rigidity*

- It occurs especially in cases of:
  A - Sudden **A**sphyxial death
  B - Injury to the **B**rain
  C - **C**erebral hemorrhage
  D - **D**rowning, **D**i nitro ortho cresol poisoning
  E - **E**xhaustion
  F - **F**ear, **F**irearm injury.

76. Legal age at which foetus is capable of independent existence:

A. 240 days **B.** 230 days
C. 220 days **D.** 210 days

74. D **75. C** **76. D**

Concept:

Viability: Physical ability of a fetus to lead "separate existence".
A child is legally viable after 210 days (7 × 30 days).
Memory cue–> count down 2-1-0-viable.

77. A bullet fired from a gun is not released. It is ejected out with the subsequent shot. It is known as:
- **A.** Dumbum bullet
- **B.** Rocketing bullet
- **C.** Ricochet bullet
- **D.** Tandem bullet

78. Brown-coloured urine is seen in the:
- **A.** Nitric acid poisoning
- **B.** Carbolic acid poisoning
- **C.** Hydrochloric and poisoning
- **D.** Sulphuric acid poisoning

Concept:

In concentrated form nitric acid combines with organic matter and produces a yellow discoloration of tissue due to the production of picric acid (xanthoproteic reaction). The stomach is soft, friable and ulcerated and brownish discoloration. Perforation of stomach is not common.

79. Which of the following is a non-poisonous snake?
- **A.** Viper
- **B.** Krait
- **C.** Sea snake
- **D.** Rat snake

77. D **78. A** **79. D**

80. In methyl alcohol poisoning there is CNS depression, cardiac depression and optic nerve atrophy. These effects are produced due to:

A. Formaldehyde and formic acid
B. Aceldehyde
C. Pyridine
D. Acetic acid

81. Priapism occurs in:

A. Snake bite
B. Ratti poisoning
C. Cantharides poisoning
D. Arsenic poisoning

82. Which of the following section of IPC are concerned with dowry death?

A. 300
B. 302
C. 304A
D. 304B

83. A cognizable offence signifies:

A. Imprisonment upto 2 years
B. Imprisonment upto 5 years
C. Arrest without warrant
D. Fine upto Rs. 10,000

84. Hatters shake is associated with:

A. Arsenic
B. Lead
C. Mercury
D. Copper

---

80. A 81. C 82. D 83. C 84. C

85. Dried semen on clothes can be detected by:

A. Infra red
B. Spectroscopy
C. Magnifying lens
D. Ultraviolet ray

86. A teacher slapped a girl student, she suffered from 25% hearing loss which resolved on surgery. What kind of injury this is?

A. Simple
B. Grievous
C. Dangerous
D. Punishment

Concept:

Privation means act of "depriving someone of", so anything less than 100% is privation, in this case there is 25% privation of hearing, which is permanent and can only be treated with surgery. Also we should read this with clause eight, which says that any hurt which causes the sufferer unable to follow his ordinary pursuit for 20 days is grievous.

It is rational to assume that a person who has 25% hearing loss, undergoing surgery would not had used his 100% ear/hearing for atleast 20 days. So the injury becomes grievous.

87. Caustic poison erodes mucosa because:

A. Hygroscopic in nature
B. It has glue like action
C. It is being programmed to stick
D. It has affinity for mucosa

Concept:

Alkalis include sodium, potassium and ammonium hydroxide and are **bases and hygroscopic in nature** thus they dissolve in water. They all contain a positive radical and a hydroxyl group. Alkalis produce a **liquefaction necrosis** when

85. D **86. B** **87. A**

they come in contact with mucosa and penetrate deeply with full thickness burns common.

Acids cause coagulation necrosis; an eschar forms, limiting further damage. Acids tend to affect the stomach more than the esophagus.

Alkalis (more damage than acids) cause rapid liquefaction necrosis; no eschar forms, and damage continues until the alkali is neutralized or diluted. Alkalis tend to affect the esophagus more than the stomach, but ingestion of large quantities severely affects both.

88. Features of antemortem burn are all *except:*

A. Vesicle with hyperaemic base
B. Red line
C. Vesicle with air
D. Vital reaction present

89. Digitalis toxicity seen in all *except:*

A. Hyperkalemia
B. Hypomagnesemia
C. Hypercalcemia
D. Renal failure

Concept:

All hypo like hypomagnesemia, hypokalemia, hypo-renal function (renal insufficiency), hypoxemia, hypothyroidism, hypo-coronary supply (myocardial ischemia or infarction) increases digitalis toxicity. **Only calcium is hyper in the list of digitalis toxicity inducing agents.**

90. Difference between antemortem and postmortem bruise all *except*:

A. Sharp edge
B. Coagulation in blood vessels
C. Raised
D. Color change

88. C **89. A** **90. A**

Concept:

A bruise produced during live shows:
1. Swelling.
2. Colour changes (If the person survives for some time).
3. Coagulation (Clotting) of the extravasated blood in the subcutaneous tissues and muscle fibres. These signs are absent if the bruise is produced after death.

91. Formication and delusion of persecution occurs in:
A. Cocaine
B. Amphetamine
C. Cannabis
D. Morphine

Concept:

Tactile hallucination is common in cocaine psychosis. This may take the form of small ants crawling over the body socalled formication. In cocaine psychosis this type of hallucination occurs together with delusion of persecution and is known as cocaine bug.

92. A farm worker presented with abdominal pain with garlic odour and linear line in nails:
A. Lead poisoning B. Arsenic
C. Mercury D. Copper

Concept:

Arsenic Poisoning:
Garlicky odor on breath; Hyperkeratosis, Rain-drop hyperpigmentation, **Black Foot,** Exfoliative dermatitis and Mees lines (transverse white striae of the fingernails); Sensory and motor polyneuritis, Distal weakness, Radiopaque sign on abdominal X-ray, ECG QRS broadening, QT prolongation, ST depression, T-wave flattening.

91. A **92. B**

93. Cuts on genitalia:

A. Homicidal **B.** Suicidal
C. Accidental **D.** Self inflicted

Concept:

Incised wounds on ears, nose, genitalia are invariably homicidal in nature. Cuts on genitalia may be result of sexual jealousy, caused by angry paramour, husband or wife.

94. Bruise are most prominent with minimum force is seen in:

A. Scalp **B.** Soles
C. Palm **D.** Face

95. Allopurinol is used in organ preservative as:

A. Free radical scavenger
B. Antioxidant
C. Preservative
D. None

Concept:

Organ Preservatives and Functions

Preservatives	*Category*	*Function*
Lactobionate, raffinose, citrate, gluconate	Osmotic active agents	Prevent cell swelling
Na+, K+, Ca+, Mg+	Electrolytes	Exert an osmotic effect
Phosphate, histidine, N -(2-hydroxyethyl)-piperazine- N'-2-ethanesulfonic acid (HEPES) buffer	H+ ion buffers	Regulate extracellular H+
Albumin, HES	Colloid	Initial vascular flush out and perfusion
Allopurinol, antiproteases, chlorpromazine	Metabolic inhibitors	Suppresses degradation of cell constituents by scavenging free radicals
Adenosine, glutathione	Metabolites	Facilitate restoration of metabolism on reperfusion
Amino steroids, Vitamin E, deferoxamine (Desferal)	Antioxidants	Inhibit oxygen free-radical injury

93. A **94. D** **95. A**

96. Destructive power of bullet is determined by:

A. Velocity **B.** Size
C. Shape **D.** Weight

Concept:

External Ballistics from Gun to Target

The external ballistics of a bullet's path can be determined by several formulae, the simplest of which is:

Kinetic Energy (KE) = 1/2 MV^2

Velocity plays a much larger role than Weight, Size and Shape in destruction caused at the target. Higher the kinetic energy more destructive power.

97. All are traumatic asphyxia *except:*

A. Railway accident
B. Road traffic accident
C. Accidental strangulation
D. Stampede

98. Extensive abrasions are found on the body of a pedestrian lying by the roadside. What is the cause?

A. Primary impact injury
B. Secondary impact injury
C. Secondary injury
D. Postmortem artifact

Concept:

Pedestrian Injuries:

1. **Primary impact injuries:** These are caused when first part of the body strikes the vehicle. In the typical case, the victim is struck by the front of the vehicle and sustains socalled bumper injury on legs.

---

96. A **97.** C **98.** C

2. **Secondary impact injuries:** These are injuries caused by further impact by the vehicle.
3. **Tertiary impact injuries (Secondary injuries):** These injuries are caused when the victim striking objects such as the ground resulting in extensive abrasions.

99. Privileged communication:

A. Doctor and patient
B. Doctor and another doctor
C. Doctor and law enforcement authorities
D. Doctor and paramedics

100. Fingerprints are destroyed in:

A. Syphilis
B. Contact dermatitis
C. Leprosy
D. Electrocution

101. Stellate wound is caused at:

A. Contact range
B. Close range
C. Intermediate range
D. Long range

102. Ant bite resembles:

A. Abrasion
B. Bruise
C. Incised wound
D. Lacerations

[N.B.: All the Questions could be answered from the 4th Edition of Review of Forensic Medicine with 100% Strike Rate!]

103. What is Falanga?

A. Beating on soles with blunt object
B. Plucking hairs
C. Persistent pushing of head into vomit
D. Beating on soles

99. C 100. C 101. A 102. A 103. A

Concept:

Methods of Torture

1. **Telefona** consists of repeated slapping of the sides of the head [over the ears] by open palms of the assailant. This may **cause rupture of ear drums**.
2. **Falanga** also known as falaka or bastinado. In this canes/rods are used to beat on the soles of the feet, which is very painful and debilitating. Aseptic necrosis may occur. Also hyperpigmentation is seen along lines of injury.
3. **Submarino** [also known as latina] victim suffers forced immersion of head in water often contaminated with feces/urine until suffocation.
4. **Dry Submarino** is tying a plastic bag over the head upto the point of suffocation.
5. **Saw Horse** forced straddling of a bar, forcing the victim to sit on a rod like one sits on horse back, leading to perineal/scrotal hematoma.
6. **Cattle Prod** [electric shock] here a magnetic device delivering high voltage may be used in which burns may not be found on skin, but it causes severe pain.
7. **Black Slave** here a heated metal spear like object, is inserted into anus causing rectal/perinea burns.

104. Hydrocution refers to:

A. Drowning in cold water
B. Electrocution in water
C. Postmortem immersion
D. Immersion in boiling water

105. Not a constituent of embalming fluid:

A. Phenol **B.** Ethanol
C. Formalin **D.** Glycerine

104. A **105. C**

Concept:

Embalming: Typically embalming fluid contains a mixture of formaldehyde, methanol, ethanol and other solvents. The formaldehyde content generally ranges from 5 to 29 percent and the ethanol content may range from 9 to 56 percent. The process of embalming is designed to slow the decomposition of the body.

Potential Ingredients include:

a. **Preservative:** 18%-35% mixture of formaldehyde, glutaraldehyde or in some cases phenol which are then diluted to gain the final index of the arterial solution. Methanol is used to hold the formaldehyde in solution. **Formalin refers specifically to 37% aqueous formaldehyde and is not commonly used in funeral embalming but rather in the preservation of anatomical specimens.**

b. **Water Conditioner:** These are designed to balance the "hardness" of water (the presence of other trace chemicals that changes the water's pH or neutrality). Additionally, water conditioners may be used to help "inactivate" chemotherapy drugs and antibiotics which may bind to and render ineffectual the preservative chemical.

c. **Cell Conditioner:** These chemicals act to prepare cells for absorption of arterial fluid and help break up clots in the bloodstream.

d. **Dyes:** Active dyes are used to restore someone's natural colouration and countersta in against conditions such as jaundice as well as to indicate distribution of arterial fluid. Inactive dyes are used by the manufacturer of the arterial fluid to give a pleasant color to the fluid in the bottle, but does nothing for the appearance of the embalmed body.

e. **Humectants:** These are added to dehydrated and emaciated bodies to help restore tissue to a more natural and hydrated appearance. These are hygroscopic substance. Examples of humectants include glycerin, propylene glycol and glyceryl triacetate. Others can be polyols like sorbitol, xylitol and maltitol, or polymeric polyols like polydextrose or natural extracts like quillaia, or lactic acid or urea. Lithium chloride is an excellent humectant but is toxic.

f. **Anti-Edemic Chemicals:** The opposite of humectants these are designed to draw excessive fluid (edema) from a body.

g. **Additional Disinfectants:** For certain cases, such as tissue gas, specialist chemicals normally used topically such as dis-spray are added to an arterial solution.

h. **Water:** Most arterial solutions are a mix of some of the preceding chemicals with tepid water. Cases done without the addition of water are referred to specifically as "waterless". Waterless embalming is very effective but not economically viable for everyday cases.

i. **Cavity Fluid:** This is generally a very high index formaldehyde or glutaraldehyde solution injected undiluted directly via the trocar incision into the body cavities to treat the viscera. In cases of tissue gas phenol based products are often used instead. Phenol, also known as **carbolic acid,** is used chiefly in cavity fluid formulations.

106. Thanatology is study of:

A. Death
B. Pollen grains
C. Dead newborn
D. Postmortem interval

---

106. A

107. A man working as a pest killer comes to OPD with pain in abdomen and garlic odour in breath with transverse line on nails poisoning is due to:

A. Lead B. Arsenic
C. Mercury D. Cadmium

108. Corpus delicti is meaning:

A. Essence of crime
B. Inquest into death
C. Body of victim
D. Postmortem examination

109. Irresistible sexual desire in a male is otherwise known as:

A. Nymphomania B. Tribadism
C. Satyriasis D. Sadism

110. In asphyxia structure to be open last is: (N.B. To obtain bloodless field neck is opened last).

A. Head B. Neck
C. Abdomen D. Thorax

111. Fingerprint Bureau was 1st established in:

A. India B. UK
C. USA D. Poland

112. Corporobasal index is used to determine:

A. Race B. Sex
C. Age D. Stature

113. Which of the following is not a death due to suffocation?

A. Burking B. Gagging
C. Throttling D. Choking

---

107. B **108. A** **109. C** **110. B** **111. A**
112. B **113. C**

114. On postmortem examination, contusion of neck muscles is seen along with fracture of hyoid bone. The most probable cause of death is:
A. Manual strangulation
B. Drowning
C. Burking
D. Smothering

115. Expanded lungs may sink due to:
A. Atelectasis
B. Putrefaction
C. Mouth to mouth respiration
D. Alcoholic fixation meconium aspiration

116. The reagent used to detect presence of vaginal cells on the penis of an accused in a rape case is:
A. Lugol's iodine
B. Phenophthalein test
C. Orthotoluidine test
D. Benzidine

Concept:

Vaginal cells cannot be seen with the naked eye, but can be detected by a test. These cells turn **Brown when exposed to the vapors of Lugol's iodine**.

117. Mechanism of labour in abortion stick is due to:
A. Stimulation of uterine contraction
B. Oxytocin present in the stick
C. Prostaglandins present in the stick
D. All of the above

118. An example of polychlorinated hydrocarbon is:
A. Parathion B. Malathion
C. Diazinon D. Endrin

114. A 115.A 116. A 117. A 118. D

119. A middle aged man from West Bengal presents with paraesthesia of hands and feet, hyperkeratosis, lines in the nails and rain drop pigmentation in the hands. The most likely causative toxin for the above mentioned symptoms is:

A. Lead
B. Arsenic
C. Thallium
D. Mercury

120. Telefona:

A. Plucking hairs
B. Beating on both ears
C. Persistent pushing of head into vomit
D. Beating on soles

121. Primary impact injury most commonly involved is:

A. Head **B.** Neck
C. Abdomen **D.** Legs

122. In death due to asphyxia, last to be opened is:

A. Thorax **B.** Abdomen
C. Head **D.** Neck

123. In tandem bullet the number of bullets fired are:

A. 1 **B.** 2
C. 3 **D.** None

124. All of the following are included in grievous hurt *except*:

A. Abrasion on face
B. Loss of one kidney
C. Loss of one testis
D. Loss of one eye

---

119. B 120. B 121. D 122. D
123. B 124. A

125. According to Nysten's Rule, the correct sequence of appearance of rigor mortis is:

A. Eyelids - Neck- Thorax - Upper Limb
B. Face- Neck- Upper limb- Thorax
C. Orbicularis Occuli - Face- Neck - Upper Limb
D. Orbicularis Occuli - Face - Upper Limb- Thorax

(Flip to Chapter 2 on Rigor Mortis)

126. Match the given Declarations with their respective intended purposes:

A. Declaration of Oslo	i. Abortion
B. Declaration of Tokyo	ii. Hippocratic oath
C. Declaration of Helsinki	iii. Human experimentation
D. Declaration of Geneva	iv. Torture

(a) A-i, B-ii, C-iii, D-iv
(b) A-iv, B-iii, C-ii, D-i
(c) A-i, B-iv, C-iii, D-ii
(d) A-ii, B-iii, C-iv, D-i

127. Atropine is not an antidote in:

A. TIK 20
B. Endrin
C. Baygone spray
D. Parathion

Concept:

Atropine is used as antidote for organophosphorous compounds but atropine is given as antidote until the tracheobronchial secretions stops.

Endrin is organochlorides which dilates the pupils.
Other OCs - Dieldrin, Aldrin, DDT, Lindane.

125. A 126. C 127. B

128. Match the following:

A. Capsicum	i. White lady
B. Croton tiglium	ii. Hunan hand
C. Cocaine	iii. Breaking bad
D. Methamphetamine	iv. Jamalghota

(a) A-ii, B-iv, C-i, D-iii
(b) A-i, B-iv, C-iii, D-ii
(c) A-ii, B-iv, C-iii, D-i
(d) A-iv, B-i, C-ii, D-iii

129. What are Borges lines?

A. Lines of fracture in mosaic fracture of bone
B. Lines of pressure in a bone due to bullet projectile
C. Lines of redness around wound after healing
D. Relaxed tension lines in skin

Concept:

- **Kraissl's lines** are a set of anatomical skin lines, these lines are oriented perpendicular to the action of the underlying muscles.
- **Langer's lines (Cleavage lines):** Generally parallel to the orientation of the underlying muscle fibres. Wounds against Langer's lines has more scarring compared to those along these lines.
- **Borges lines:** Follow the relaxed skin tension lines.
- **Blaschko**, are lines of normal cell development in the skin.
- The Kraissl's lines correspond to the movements of the skin during muscle work and the Borges lines are the relaxed skin tension lines.

128. A 129. D

130. All are correct *except*:

A. Upper third molar is most commonly absent in Mongolians

B. Caucasians have carabelli cusps

C. In Negroes the cusps of molars are wide and deep and shovel shaped cusps in incisors

D. Prominent lingual ridge and labial ridge in Mongols

Concept:

Flip to Chapter 1 on Teeth and Race.

131. Causes of death in prolonged Jack knife position is due to:

A. Burking

B. Traumatic asphyxia

C. Positional asphyxia

D. Wedging

Concept:

Positional asphyxia is mostly accident-associated with alcohol or drug intoxication. Individuals get trapped in restricted spaces or get into unusual positions like Jack Knife position.

N.B.→ Q. 125–131 were asked in 2017 All India Institute of Medical Sciences – Pre PG Exams.

130. C **131.** C

17

The Forensic Name Game

Assignment for Readers

(a) Correlate with corresponding chapters and put a ***handwritten note*** there, for high memory yield.
(b) Add more ***eponyms*** here which you discover during the course of your study.
(c) Frequently gauge your preparation strategy with this litmus test:

"Read Less, Study More"

1. **Ashley's Rule of 149:** Ashley formulated the "149 rule", according to which a male **sternum** exceeded 149 mm in length, whereas the female sternum was less than 149 mm.
2. **Barr body for Sex Determination:** It is the inactive X chromosome in a female somatic cell, rendered inactive in a process called **lionization.**
3. **Bertillon's system of Anthropometry:** Alphonse Bertillon used photography and measurement to create a record of unique **identifiers** that could be used to track suspects, inmates and repeat offenders.
4. **Burtonion line of Pb:** A stippled blue colored line present in upper jaw due to lead-sulphide at the junction of the teeth and gums (Pb is pB →lead).

5. **Beckwith's Sign of SIDS:** Reduced number or a complete absence of petechial hemorrhages in the rear upper part of the **Thymus** over the course of the brachiocephalic vein in **Sudden Infant Death Syndrome (SIDS).**
   Explanation: *Local protective role of the brachiocephalic vein prior to changes in intrathoracic pressure.*
6. **Carbelli's Cusps** seen in white races, used in identification (see Chapter 1).
7. **Casper's Dictum of Putrefaction:** The speed ratio of human body putrefaction in the air, in water and underground (approximately 8:2:1).
   Explanation: *The differences in the speed of putrefactive changes are based on the* ***dissimilar amount of oxygen*** *in the air, water and underground.*
8. **'Devonshire Colic':** A condition that affected people in Devon during parts of the 17th and 18th centuries before it was discovered to be lead poisoning.
9. **Duret's (Henri) Hemorrhages of Brainstem:** These are small lineal areas of bleeding in the midbrain and upper pons of the brainstem, delayed secondary hemorrhages due to increased intracranial pressure–caused by a traumatic downward displacement of the brainstem.
10. **Ewing's Postulates:** In order to prove the existence of a causal relation of **trauma to cancer,** Dr. James Ewing has established minimal criteria (see Chapter 4).
11. **Gustafson's Method of Age:** The age estimation of adult over 25 years (between 25 and 60 years) depends on the physiological age changes in each of the dental tissue–Postmortem Method.
12. **Greulich and Pyle Atlas:** Age estimation from bones (see Chapter 1).
13. ***Haase's Formula of Fetal Age:*** Karl Friedrich Haase's formula for suggesting the age of a human fetus or newborn from its length.

14. **Henssge Nomogram (HN)** is used for calculating time of death based on body temperature measurement (Algor Mortis).
15. **Kennedy's Phenomenon of Surgical Artefact:** Due to surgical alteration evaluation of wound as entry or exit wound becomes difficult.
16. **Kevorkian Sign of Retinal Blood Column Segmentation:** Continuous blood column in the retinal blood vessels breaks up into small segments, which then collide with each other. This looks like movement of wagons of railway train, hence the term rail-roading phenomenon. ***Explanation:*** *Rapid fall in blood pressure and shrinkage of fibrin in the clotted blood in the retinal vessels.*
17. **Krogman's Table* of Sexing:** Percentage of accuracy in determination of sex from bone.
18. **Krønlein's Shot of Firearm:** Brain evisceration of a gunshot wound to the head by a military rifle.
    Explanation: *Prolapse of an intact brain hemisphere or both brain hemispheres in high velocity missile injuries to the brain.*
19. **Lichtenberg's Flowers of Lightning:** Specific branching pattern found in solid materials when exposed to high voltage levels. Also called Lightning figures or **KeraUnoGraphic signs**.
    Explanation: *Lightning injuries inflicted by **high voltage lightning** or electric shock. Skin lesions in the form of tree-like reddish-brown patterns arranged on the surface of the skin. It is due to **Paralysis of Capillaries** and **Thermal Denaturation of Erythrocytes**. These figures disappear after 24 hours, if victim survives.*
20. **Marshall's Triad of Explosion Injuries:** Marshall's triad includes punctate-bruises, abrasions and small punctate lacerations all of

which are typically found in an explosive bomb blast.

21. **Megnin's 8 Waves of Forensic Entomology:** Megnin recognized that the colonisation of corpses in air by different species of insects takes place in **8 predictable waves**; his book "La faune des cadavres" published in 1894 is a milestone of the forensic entomology.

22. **Nysten's Law of Rigor Mortis:** Postmortem muscle stiffness, proceeds from the head downwards, in Cranio→Caudal direction.

    Explanation: *The stiffness first develops in masticatory muscles→facial and neck muscles→Upper and lower extremities also known as* ***"Descendent".***

23. **Paltauf's Spots (Also known as Rasskazov-Lukomskij Spots) of Drowning:** Petechial hemorrhages located beneath the pulmonary pleura in both lungs, and appear in wet drowning.

    [N.B.→Paltauf's spots are larger and not as sharply defined due to hemolysis as in case of Tardieau's Spots].

24. **Puppe's Rule of Fracture lines:** Helps to determine the **Sequence of Bullets** in multiple bullet injuries in skull.

    Explanation: *Fracture lines created by every other shot extend only up to the fractured lines produced by the previous shot(s) without crossing over previously created fracture line.*

25. **Quetelet's Rule* of biological variation:** Applicable to variation in Fingerprints.

26. **Raekillo Classical Study** of histochemical changes in wounds, to estimate time of injury.

27. **Sehrt's Sign of Drowning:** Microruptures of **Gastric Mucosa** are considered a secondary corroborative finding in **Wet Drowning.**

    Explanation: *These microruptures are arranged radially and found mainly at the* *lesser curvature of the stomach. Their formation is due to **the stretching of the stomach** due to the swallowed liquid or water.*

28. **Simon's Sign of Spine:** Hemorrhages in intervertebral discs beneath the anterior longitudinal ligament in the intervertebral discs of the lower thoracic and lumbar typically seen in **hanging**.
Explanation: Rostro-caudal elongation of the spine due to the neck's suspension in the noose, agonal spasms, and decorticate rigidity with extension of the trunk and lower extremities. They may also occur in non-asphyxia hyperextensive spinal injuries.
29. **Stack's Method of Infant Age:** Stack evolved a method to know the age of infants from the weight and height of the erupting **teeth of child.**
30. **Sveshnikov's Sign of Drowning:** Seen in wet drowning and indicates the presence of free liquid in the maxillary and sphenoid paranasal sinuses.
31. **Taner and Whitehouse Method** of estimation of age from bone X-rays.
32. **Tardieu's Spots:** Ecchymosis or petechial hemorrhages beneath the pulmonary and parietal pleura developing in mechanical asphyxia. They can also be found beneath the epicardium and thymus capsule. It forms part of '**Visceral Congestion Syndrome**', also known as **Bayard's Ecchymoses.**
33. **Washburn Index:** Ischium-Pubis Index used in sex determination.
34. **Wischnewski Spots (of hypothermia):** Petechial hemorrhages and erosions in the gastric and duodenal mucosa is characteristic of death due to hypothermia. These are erosions of ectopic gastric mucosa in the esophagus or small intestine seen in 40–90% of hypothermia cases.

35. **Wydler's Sign of Wet Drowning:** Auxiliary diagnostic autopsy sign of Wet Drowning, i.e., Foamy, liquid stomach content of a drowned person. This sign typically consists of 3 basic components:
    (i) Foam on the top.
    (ii) Liquid in the middle; and
    (iii) Solid component at the bottom.

18

*The Forensic Imaginarium**

In Pre-PG Exams many image based questions are being asked these days including in Forensic Medicine. In order to answer such questions, it is important to know the standard topics in each chapter, from which image based questions could be asked. Instead of printing multiple images within each chapter and making this book thicker, static and costlier, I've created a closed Facebook Group called **"#RoFM Forensic Imaginarium"**. The Group will be 3D – **Digital, Discussion based and Dynamic.**

The purpose of the FB Group is two folds:

(a) Equipping students to prepare for image based questions.

(b) Revising Forensic Medicine in a vivid manner for greater retention.

Join the Facebook Group*   **§§ #RoFM Forensic Imaginarium §§**   https://www.facebook.com/groups/ForensicImaginarium/

* For Current Owners of **'Review of Forensic Medicine'** + Future ones!

Potential Question Zones – for Image Based Questions and Rapid Revision

I. Identification

Shape of skulls| Fragmented Medulla| Barr Body, Davidson-Smith Body| Male vs Female Pelvis|

Charting of Teeth – Palmer Notation, Universal System| X-Rays showing Fusion of Joints| Osteometric Board and Stature| Fingerprints – identifying loops, whorls[NEET], Arches, Delta, Core, Recurve| Tattoo Mark| Unique shape of the frontal sinuses|

II. Thanatology

Taches noires de Sclerotica| Graphs of progression of Algor Mortis, Livor Mortis, and Rigor Mortis| Henssge nomogram| Cadaveric Spasm| Postmortem Lividity–Blanching and Fixed lividity| Drowning victim clutching vegetation| Decomposition – earliest change green discoloration of the lower right abdominal quadrant| Miliaria seen in advance decomposition| Marbling| Postmortem Blisters| Putrefaction with Skin Slippage| Adipocere| Mummification| Postmortem Purge| Postmortem Ant bite marks with NO vital tissue reaction| Postmortem Artefacts.

III. Injuries and Its Medicolegal Importance

Abrasions–especially Patterned Abrasions, Tyre marks| Bite Mark leading to symmetrical abrasions| Contusions–Railway (Tram) Track bruising, Ectopic bruising, Battle's Sign, Racoon sign| Grey-Turner's Sign, bruising of the abdominal flanks| Cullen's sign: Bruising around Umbilicus – Intraperitoneal Haemorrhage|

Incised wounds – Hesitation parallel marks| Lacerations – Incised Looking Lacerated wounds, Tissue Bridges, Avulsion laceration| Stab wounds–Fish Tailing seen in single edge weapon| Dicing injuries and Sparrow's foot mark – wind shield injuries | Wedge shaped bumper fracture of Tibia/Fibula| Fracture Skull – types| Signature – Depressed Fracture| Intracranial Haemorrhage–types| Duret haemorrhages in midbrain| Fat Embolism Syndrome – Pinpoint blood spots in white matter|

Firearm wounds–diagram of a cartridge, calibre, Entry wound, Exit wound, Abrasion collar, Puppe's Rule| Stippling (but no soot) intermediate range firearms| Contact Entry wound on forehead – showing stellate shape| Blast Injuries – Marshall's triad, Blast lungs.

IV. Toxicology

Arsenic – Rain Drop Pigmentations, Mee's Lines| Lead – Burtonion's Line| Mercury – Acrodynia, Pink's Disease| Dhatura Seeds vs Capsicum seeds| 'Foam cone' seen with narcotic overdoses| Abrus – Suis–cattle poison–resembles snake bite| Histology Slide showing calcium oxalate renal crystals – Ethylene Glycol Poisoning |

V. Violent Asphyxial Deaths

Atypical Hanging| Ligature Marks| Conjunctival petechial haemorrhage| Tardieu's Spots | Le facies sympathique| Dribbling of Saliva| Fracture Hyoid Bone – Inward compression vs Anteroposterior fracture| Garrotting| Throttling – extensive bruising inside, no ligature mark| Drowning – Froth, Cadaveric Spasm clutching the straws and grass, Washer woman's Hands, Cutis Anserina, Paltauf's haemorrhages, Emphysema aquosum, Diatoms, histology of drowned lungs|

VI. Infanticide is Murder

Maceration – Skin discoloration and slippage, darkened umbilical cord | Robert's sign | Battered Baby Syndrome| String of Beads appearance on X- Rays| On autopsy the skull bone is opened using a 'rose-petal' or 'butterfly' method.

VII. Thermal Injuries

Wischnewski ulcers are superficial gastric mucosal erosions seen in Hypothermia | Puppet Organs| Soot particles in trachea – antemortem burns| Pugilistic attitude both antemortem and postmortem burns | Heat Ruptures| Joule Burn| Crocodile skin lesions| Nuclear streaming on histology is seen in electrical injuries| Lightening Injuries – Filligree burns|

Epilogue

> Most murderers make the mistake of spending too much time planning to commit a murder; and too less on how to dispose! the body. – s.s

Many students spend most of their time reading multiple books, notes, running after more and more facts, information, and less on how to dispose! already acquired study material. The secret of success is not in reading more but in studying more. Revision helps to catalogue study material within the deep recesses of mind in a way that can be retrieved easily during the exam. Revision slows down forgetting.

Context Dependent Memory: Studying – at the same place, at the same study desk, facing the same direction, under similar circumstances – helps to establish a vivid context in which a topic was studied. This works at two levels. One, it slowly conditions the mind to get into 'study groove' as soon as one is in a familiar study environment. This enhances the efficiency while studying. Two, retrieval of information is greatly facilitated when one vividly remembers the surroundings in which the information was assimilated. This is called context dependent memory.

Using Imagery for High Yield: Try translating words into images by either drawing schematic diagrams, sketches of cognitive maps or simply taking cryptic notes. This will help in active processing of the study material and convert abstract concepts into concrete retrievable structures. Images last longer in mind than mere words and thus help in faster revision.

Before concluding let me reiterate what I said. Always study in the same place and preferably during the same time slots. Always write, draw, sketch, or at least scribble concepts, facts, cognitive maps while one reads and then revise them.

Revision is more powerful than plain reading. That is, how "Read less, Study more" works – always.

